A History of Women in Medicine and Medical Research

For Erin.
All I've Ever Needed.

A History of Women in Medicine and Medical Research

Exploring the Trailblazers of STEM

Dale DeBakcsy

PEN & SWORD
HISTORY
AN IMPRINT OF PEN & SWORD BOOKS LTD.
YORKSHIRE – PHILADELPHIA

First published in Great Britain in 2022 by
PEN AND SWORD HISTORY
An imprint of
Pen & Sword Books Ltd
Yorkshire – Philadelphia

ISBN 978 1 39906 896 3

A CIP catalogue record for this book is available from the British Library.

Typeset in Times New Roman 11/13.5 by
SJmagic DESIGN SERVICES, India.
Printed and bound in the UK by CPI Group (UK) Ltd.

Pen & Sword Books Limited incorporates the imprints of Atlas, Archaeology, Aviation, Discovery, Family History, Fiction, History, Maritime, Military, Military Classics, Politics, Select, Transport, True Crime, Air World, Frontline Publishing, Leo Cooper, Remember When, Seaforth Publishing, The Praetorian Press, Wharncliffe Local History, Wharncliffe Transport, Wharncliffe True Crime and White Owl.

For a complete list of Pen & Sword titles please contact
PEN & SWORD BOOKS LIMITED
47 Church Street, Barnsley, South Yorkshire, S70 2AS, England
E-mail: enquiries@pen-and-sword.co.uk
Website: www.pen-and-sword.co.uk

PEN AND SWORD BOOKS
1950 Lawrence Rd, Havertown, PA 19083, USA
E-mail: Uspen-and-sword@casematepublishers.com
Website: www.penandswordbooks.com

FSC www.fsc.org
MIX
Paper | Supporting responsible forestry
FSC® C013604

Contents

Introduction

Women have been practising medicine from deepest antiquity. In the twenty-seventh century BCE, Peseshet, an Egyptian physician of the fourth or fifth Dynasty, carried the title 'lady overseer of female physicians'. The Sumerians, before their absorption by the more misogynistic Akkadian Empire in the twenty-fourth century BCE, employed female physicians as a matter of course. Like their male counterparts, they were denoted by shaved heads. The ancient Greeks recorded Laïs, Aspasia, Elephantis and Metrodora as famous medical practitioners, the last of whose text, *On the Diseases and Cures of Women,* ranks as the earliest surviving text written by a woman about women's medicine.

Women continued to be well represented in medicine throughout the Middle Ages, from noble women who used their position and resources to found and administer hospitals, to the leaders of religious orders who expanded the activities of their institutions to include the medical care of the poor and needy. In the twelfth century, Italy became a world centre for the training and advancement of women physicians, with Salerno in particular serving as a capital of women's medical practice until roughly the fifteenth century. Here, for a few shining centuries, women obtained university medical educations, taught and demonstrated in higher institutions, saw patients of both genders suffering from every manner of malady, and wrote streams of medical treatises that recalled the achievements of their counterparts in Greco-Roman antiquity.

The success of the Italian women physicians was replicated, though encumbered with more official restrictions, in France and Spain during the late Middle Ages, particularly with the need for trained medical personnel occasioned by the fourteenth-century outbreak of plague, but later, women physicians experienced a precipitous downfall in numbers as medicine professionalised itself in the early Modern era. Once a university education became a prerequisite for the practice of medicine, women were pushed into peripheral services such as the creation of medications and the practice of midwifery, before those professions were in turn cracked down upon by a now male-dominated medical establishment increasingly unwilling to brook competition.

By the nineteenth century, the preparation of medicine, delivery of children, practice of family medicine, and performance of surgery all lay firmly in the hands of a professionalised male community of practitioners whose financial self-interest aligned perfectly with the cultural concerns of a Victorian society that believed it would be the ruin of women to learn about the functioning of the human body. Beginning in the 1840s, individual women challenged the admissions criteria of particular universities in an increasingly coordinated attempt to open the gates of education, resulting in the prestigious Zurich University opening its doors to women students in 1864, followed shortly by the Sorbonne admitting women to its secondary education lectures in 1867.

Meanwhile, in the United States, the solution to the problem of women's medical education was found at first not in the opening of prestigious men's institutions, but in the creation of new colleges specifically for women. The New England Female Medical College (1848) and Female Medical College of Pennsylvania (1850) represented early small-scale attempts to offer medical instruction to women, but students soon realised that education was nothing without a place to practise their trade. They needed experience to hone their knowledge, and without any hospitals willing to accept them as interns, it was up to enterprising women to create their own hospitals. Soon the New York Infirmary for Indigent Women and Children (founded in 1857 by Elizabeth Blackwell) and the New England Hospital for Women and Children (founded in 1862 by Blackwell's associate Marie Zakrzewska) were attracting women the world over who would go on to create similar institutions in their home countries.

The late nineteenth century represented the high-water mark of the women's medical college and women's hospital movement, born of necessity and kept alive by institutional inertia. Yale Medical did not admit women until 1916; Harvard Medical did not accept its first woman student until 1945. While Oxford allowed women to attend classes in the 1870s, they were not allowed to take full degrees for their work until 1920 and Cambridge, not to be outdone in the realm of academic heel-dragging, though it let women sit for exams as early as 1882, did not award women full university degrees until 1948! And yet, though the larger institutions took their time bowing to the inevitable progress of civilisation, sufficient smaller universities began opening their doors throughout the late nineteenth and early twentieth century that the women's colleges were either slowly absorbed by larger co-educational institutions (as the New England Female Medical College was absorbed into Boston University in 1874) or closed their doors completely (as Sophia Jex-Blake's Edinburgh School of Medicine for Women did in 1898).

Having been for millennia a regular presence in the medical profession, and for a few centuries a complete absence therein, by the mid-1950s women had finally clawed their way back to a theoretical equality of educational opportunity. In practice, however, as we shall come to see, women were routinely discouraged from taking those opportunities, either by faculties who were unwilling to entertain the costly training of a doctor who was just going to, so the theory went, abandon her profession at the first opportunity to have children, or by educational structures that did not, until the revolutionary efforts of Mary Bunting in the 1960s, adjust the configuration of departmental expectations to meet the unique needs of women students.

Today, new waves of women medical students are finally putting a dent in gender inequities three centuries in the making. In 2019, the Association of American Medical Colleges reported that women made up 50.5 per cent of the medical students in the nation, a trend which should, in the coming decades, improve the representation of women among full professors (a dismal 21 per cent by a 2016 AAMC reckoning) and practising physicians (at 36.3 per cent as of 2019, up from 34 per cent in 2015), and return us at last to the place we were, several thousand years ago.

Chapter 1

Trota of Salerno and the Problem of Medieval Women's Medicine

Imagine it is the twelfth century, and you have woken up experiencing some trouble breathing. Fortunately, you have the financial resources to hire a top-tier, exquisitely learned physician to attend you. He listens closely to your problems, and knows at once what to do. Your uterus, he tells you, has wandered up into your chest cavity and is interfering with your lungs.

Sounds reasonable, you say, but what do we do about it?

But of course, all the great authorities are in agreement, he assures you. We simply must drive the uterus back down where it belongs by coating your nose with foul-smelling substances and burning or boiling sweet-smelling ones near your vagina. The uterus, which everybody knows has a sense of smell, will be repelled by the foul-smelling compounds, and attracted to the sweet ones, and will swim back to its proper place. Case closed.

Medieval medicine is the quintessential example of just how persuasively complicated and nuanced a body of knowledge can appear while being at the same time wrong in just about all of its assumptions and conclusions. The theories of the Hippocratic authors and the humours of the Galenic tradition filtered their way through copiers and editors on two continents, evolving into ever more learned theories about how bodies *should* work, while steadily losing contact with how they *actually* did.

For male patients, the results were unnerving enough, but for women the treatments they were subjected to ranged from the absurd but harmless to the positively barbarous. Women were entirely at the mercy of theoretical systems that used theological and philosophical ideas about women's natures to form regimens for the regulation of their bodies. Because women were considered to be dominated by 'cold' humours, it was considered necessary for the maintenance of their health to regularly eject heat through menstruation, a process which doctors would help along by slashing the soles of women's feet with scalpels or producing lesions around the genitals so as to 'pull' the body's blood downwards, and thus towards the womb.

Likewise, if a woman was menstruating *too* much and thus losing too much heat, pressure cups would be applied to her breasts so as to drive blood back upwards and away from the uterus.

Bled, prodded and pulled, women were less subjects in their treatment and more a battlefield of humours to be tamed by whatever means necessary so that procreation could proceed apace.

The only thing to be said of this long tradition was that it held a generally positive view of menstruation and sexual activity as normal, healthful and necessary. But otherwise, it was male-crafted theory that led practice until the late twelfth century when a woman physician by the name of Trota of Salerno took it upon herself to write not about what ought to work in the curing of women's diseases, but about what actually *did* work in practice. The resulting texts on the practical aspects of women's health would stand as the definitive works on the subject for three full centuries.

We know next to nothing about Trota's life story other than that she probably lived in the mid-twelfth century and came from the southern Italian city of Salerno. Those two mere facts however speak volumes, as twelfth-century Salerno was an epicentre of medieval medical reform. A trading post between Africa and Europe, Salerno was one of the first towns in Europe to benefit from the importation of Arabic medical texts.

Sometime around 1070, a physician named Alfanus invited Constantine the African to settle in Salerno and supported him in the translation of the cream of Arabic medical knowledge. The result was a cavalcade of returned Greek practice blended with African *materia medica* knowledge, culminating in his seven volume *Viaticum*, which would hold its position as a core medical text for centuries. In a short century's time, the unremarkable town of Salerno was garnering a continental reputation for the quality and learnedness of its physicians. For those of a practical turn of mind, the new cures and medicines coming from Africa could be tested side by side with traditional Italian and wider European practices, providing a way to break out of the practical stalemate of the previous centuries.

Trota appears to have been of such a practical turn of mind, and there is no better place to see that at work than in the book that solidified her position at the centre of medieval medical practice: the *Trotula*. The first thing to know about it is that it is not a single book, but rather three books that were thrown together by a succession of well-meaning editors and reworked until it was perceived to be one text written by the great and famous Trota. In fact, however, she was only responsible for one of those books, a fact we see right away when comparing her section with the other two.

The first section, *On the Conditions of Women*, is a standard rehashing of the *Viaticum* and all its theoretical, Galenic concerns. It advises certain procedures, not because they have been observed to be effective but because they fit nicely with certain accepted intellectual tropes.

The second section, Trota's own *On Treatments for Women*, has flickers of theory here and there, but is overwhelmingly a brass tacks, 'Here's What Seems to Work', approach to women's health issues. Does your sweat stink? Bilberry leaves seem to do a pretty good job clearing that up. Are you experiencing swelling of the vagina after sex? Taking a bath infused with pennyroyal and mallow seems to help. Do you live in a restrictive society where your entire hope of happiness lies in being declared a virgin when you know perfectly well you are not one? Here are a few constrictive herbs that might help trick your prospective husband into believing you are.

The *Trotula* exists today in some 126 different manuscripts spread over four centuries, indicating that it was one of the most widely distributed medical texts of the Middle Ages, its original Latin eventually translated into Dutch, German and French. For issues relating to gynaecology, it was simply *the* reference work to have. Though it was Trota's most influential book, it was far from her most comprehensive. *Practical Medicine According to Trota* included seventy-one remedies covering both women's and men's illnesses, but it exists today in only two manuscripts, while a greater work still we know only through excerpts included in the compendium *On the Treatment of Illnesses*. That she, a woman physician, was included in that compendium on the strength of her medical reputation, without seemingly a second thought, speaks not only to her influence but to the greater possibility that women physicians were more prevalent in medieval times than we generally believe.

That we do not have Trota's complete body of works, and only know of her as a living person through one anecdote in the *Trotula* which narrates an incident when she used her level-headed knowledge of women's issues to save a female patient from the theoretically muddled ministrations of a male colleague, is deeply frustrating. There are hints and whispers in the historical record of other Salernitan women boasting both medical knowledge and a familiarity with the newly arrived corpus of African remedies, but Trota is the only named practitioner we have to grasp, examine and speculate solidly about.

That is frustrating, but at least we do have the full *Trotula*, and while I doubt anybody will be inserting a laurel-oil infused piece of lint into their vagina attached to two strings that are tied around the thighs to determine whether hot or cold humours are currently dominant in their bodies, there are moments in that book that reach across the centuries – of treating cracked lips with honey, or using hyssop to treat a coughing child, which remind us of our common humanity and deep trove of historical wisdom. Trota put practice and efficacy back at the centre of the physician's practice, a foundational step towards that grand questioning of any metaphysics masquerading as science which bloomed in the Renaissance, and flourishes still.

Further Reading

Historian Monica H. Green is perhaps the real hero of this story. She not only made the *Trotula* widely available in English for the first time with her 2001 *The Trotula: An English Translation of the Medieval Compendium of Women's Medicine*, but included in it an exhaustively researched sixty-page account of the probable authorship of the different sections of the *Trotula*, and of the twists and turns that saw three very different books gradually merged into one. She also gives a vibrant sense of what eleventh- and twelfth-century Salerno was like intellectually and commercially. It is an absolute must-have for any Women in Science collection.

Chapter 2

Brief Portraits

Women Physicians of Antiquity and the Middle Ages

Peseshet (~twenty-seventh century BCE)

Living in the Egyptian fourth Dynasty, Peseshet bore the title of 'Lady Overseer of the Female Physicians' and was therefore probably a physician herself. If you ignore the largely mythological figure of the Chinese healer Sü Nu, and the complicated case of the potentially fabricated Egyptian physician Merit Ptah, Peseshet stands as the earliest unambiguous case of a named woman physician on record.

Queen Mentuhetep (~twenty-fourth century BCE)

Mentuhetep (or Mentuhotep) is considered to have been a physician on the strength of the presence in her tomb of what is believed to be her medical kit, which contained ointment jars, measuring spoons, a mixing dish, and herbs.

Agamede (twelfth century BCE)

Sometimes known as Perimede, Agamede was a woman physician referred to by Homer in the *Iliad* as the daughter of Augeas, king of the Epeans. Homer claimed that she was a renowned expert in the healing properties of plants.

Anicia/Amyte (fourth century BCE)

According to Pausanias, Anicia was a doctor from Epidaurus who was known to perform minor operations and bleedings.

Agnodike/Agnodice (fourth century BCE/legendary)

The story of Agnodike, as told by Hyginus in his *Fabulae*, is one of the most beloved in the history of women in medicine. In it, Agnodike, in order to usefully minister to the needs of Greek women, disguised herself as a man and studied under Herophilus, a physician. When she was caught attempting to deliver a child while disguised as a male doctor, she was placed on trial, sparking an outcry from the women of Athens, which resulted in the freeing of Agnodike and the opening of the medical profession to women in Athens. It is a great story, but modern historians generally agree that it is either a complete legend, or that the story of Agnodike is an encapsulation of a larger and longer social process.

Artemisia of Caria II (fourth century BCE)

After the death of her husband, Mausolus, Artemisia took over the administration of Caria, located in Western Anatolia, personally leading her armies to victory, and ordering the construction of one of the wonders of the world, the Mausoleum at Halicarnassus, in the memory of her passed husband. She was also reputed to be an expert in herbal medicine, who discovered the herb *Artemisia* (a version of which Tu Youyou, whom we shall meet later, employed to combat malaria two millennia later) and advocated for the medicinal value of wormwood.

Laïs (second/first century BCE)

We only know about Laïs through Pliny's *Natural History*, in which she is portrayed as a midwife who was persistently at odds with the physician Elephantis over the value of different herbs and abortive treatments.

Metrodora (second/first century BCE)

Alternately believed to have lived somewhere around the third century ce, Metrodora is known as the author of the earliest known medical text penned by a woman, *On the Diseases and Cures of Women*, a thorough treatment of gynaecology in sixty-three chapters, which made new contributions on the classification of different vaginal discharges and their associated diseases.

Elephantis (first century BCE)

Mentioned by both Pliny and Galen, Elephantis was probably a physician who specialised in abortives and cosmetics, though Galen refers to her in admiration of her baldness treatments. Whether she is the same Elephantis who wrote a well-known early sex manual is at present uncertain.

Sotira (first century BCE)

Pliny rated the medicinal abilities of Sotira to treat post-partum fever as bordering on the miraculous. There is some belief that she wrote a manuscript called *Gynaeciai*, and might have lived in the first century CE rather than the first century BCE.

Aspasia the Physician (first/second century CE)

Like later medical reformer Trota of Salerno, Aspasia seems to have been a thoroughly practically minded sort of physician, who developed a useful technique for turning breech babies, and new procedures to treat uterine and scrotal swellings, which were influential for centuries.

Favilla (second century CE)

According to Galen, Favilla was a Roman physician who had developed useful remedies for diarrhoea and the coughing up of blood.

Macrina the Younger (early fourth century CE)

According to the account of Gregory of Nyssa (which, as an act of quasi-hagiography, has to be taken with a bit of salt), Macrina and her brother, Basil the Great, were responsible for the creation of a large hospital in Caesarea which had different sections for the treatment of different diseases, including a convalescent section, a section for lepers, housing for orphans and the elderly, and for the physicians and nurses who were on the staff.

Aemilia (fourth century CE)

Born in Moselle, France, Aemilia, whom we know from the writings of her nephew, the poet Ausonius, was a physician and author of texts on gynaecology

Fabiola (d. 399)

After the death of her second husband, Fabiola fell under the influence of St Jerome, who directed her to use her knowledge and energy in the service of the poor, specifically in the treatment of diseases that had caused people to become social outcasts. Towards the end of her life, she established, together with Pammachius, a former senator, a hospice for pilgrims to Rome.

Leoparda (fourth century CE)

We know of Leoparda through a book for aspiring women physicians written by Emperor Gratian's physician, Priscian Theodorus. Leoparda was one of the three women physicians of the era to whom the book was dedicated, where she is recorded as being a respected gynaecologist at Gratian's court.

Andromache (sixth century CE)

According to the *Tetrabiblion* of Aetius of Amida, Andromache was a learned physician of Aetius's era who not only knew and employed remedies from Pliny, but those she gathered from the Egyptian and Indian medical traditions as well.

Radegonde (520–587)

Forcibly wed against her will to Clotaire, the son of the French king Clovis I, the ascetic Radegonde (or Radegund) devoted her time, and her husband's resources, to the treatment of illnesses, learning from the court's physicians at first and ultimately, after fleeing her husband when he murdered her brother in a fit of rage, using her experience to establish a hospital at the convent in Poitiers which served as her refuge. Here she trained the nuns in the healing arts, and was soon treating a multitude of illnesses. In the two years following her death, the Poitiers nuns refused to accept any replacement for her as abbess.

Ælflæd (654–714)

The daughter of Oswiu, the Northumbrian king, Ælflæd was given over to Hartlepool Abbey by her father when she was 1-year-old, to be raised by an abbess by the name of Hilda, who was knowledgeable in both medicine and surgery. Hilda took Ælflæd with her when she founded Whitby Abbey in 657, and in 680, when Hilda died, Ælflæd succeeded her as abbess, and continued her tradition of using the Abbey as a centre of medical care.

Adelberger of Lombardy (eighth century)

A student of the Benedictine monk, Paul of Lombardy, Adelberger was the daughter of the Lombard king Desiderius and probably practised medicine in the middle years of the eighth century.

Agnes, Countess of Aix (fl. ~1080–~1120)

Agnes was the wife of Alard de Guillebaud until the marriage was dissolved when it was discovered how closely related Alard and Agnes were, whereupon Agnes moved to Fontevraud Abbey, which had been established by Robert of Arbrissel in 1101. In 1107, Alard donated land for a new nunnery to be founded in Orsan and Agnes became its first prioress. She was known as a healer, and ministered to Robert upon his death bed.

Agnes of Jerusalem (eleventh century)

According to Godfrey of Bouillon, the first ruler of the Kingdom of Jerusalem during the Crusades era, Agnes was a member of the Knights of St John of Jerusalem, known for providing exemplary care to wounded and sick Crusaders. Not to be confused with Agnes of Courtenay, who was also associated with the Crusader era, but lived about a century later.

Anna Komnene (1083–1148)

Anna Komnene (or Comnena) was the daughter of the Byzantine Emperor Alexios I Komnenos. She was taught Greek, astronomy, medicine, geography, mathematics and military theory by a string of private tutors, winning a reputation as one of the most brilliant women of her era. She was placed in charge of the hospital Alexios had founded in Constantinople, which reputedly had capacity for 10,000 patients. There she also taught medicine. She attempted to usurp the throne from her younger brother upon the death of her father, a coup which ultimately failed, compelling Anna to surrender her estates and ultimately retire to the convent of Kecharitomene. She was the author of a large section of the *Alexiad*, a historical account of her father's reign.

Hildegard of Bingen (1098–1179)

One of the most respected and powerful women of the Middle Ages, Hildegard is known today primarily as a musical composer, abbess and religious mystic. As a scientific thinker, we have tended to undersell her due to the visionary nature of her prose, but her works do contain both theories of the origin of the cosmos and practical descriptions of the use of plants and minerals for maintaining human health that were highly influential in their time.

Adelle of the Saracens (twelfth century)

Like Trota, Adelle was a physician active in Salerno. All we really know of her is that she was a lecturer at the Salerno Medical School.

Agnes of Bohemia (~1205–1282)

Our third Medieval Agnes was the daughter of King Ottokar I and Queen Constance of Bohemia, and as such was considered prime marriage material for the solidification of dynastic alliances. However, she turned down marriage proposals from King Henry VII of Germany, King Henry III of England, and Holy Roman Emperor Frederick II, in order to devote herself to a religious life. She built a hospital for the poor, the Hospital of St Francis, in 1232/33, and after some correspondence with Clare of Assisi, the founder of the Order of Poor Ladies, she built a monastery attached to the hospital to house the monks and nuns who worked there. She went on to found a new military order, the Knights of the Cross with the Red Star, which was devoted to the practice of nursing.

Rebecca Guarna (early thirteenth century)

One of the 'Ladies of Salerno' who carried on Trota's legacy into the thirteenth century, Rebecca Guarna studied at the University of Salerno, and was the author of *De Urinis*, *De Febrius* and *De Embrione*.

Katherine the Surgeon (thirteenth century)

Katherine is recorded as a practising physician in London, daughter of Thomas the Surgeon, who flourished sometime towards the end of the century.

Jacqueline Felice de Almania/Jacobina Felicie (b. 1280)

Felice, a Florentine physician who practised in France, is one of the best documented women doctors of the fourteenth century thanks to her 1322 trial for practising medicine without a licence. A 1220 French edict had restricted the practice of medicine to unmarried men on a Faculty of Medicine, or married men who had trained under a master. Felice had trained under a master, and was famous for taking and curing cases that her male contemporaries had given up on (and for refusing payment for treatments that did not end in a cure). But because she was a woman, the exception for having trained under a master did not apply to her, and in 1322 she was put on trial for practising medicine without a university licence, and threatened with excommunication if she resumed her practice.

Alessandra Giliani (1307–1326)

Giliani is believed to be the first recorded woman prosector. Her work involved preparing corpse dissections for the anatomical demonstrations of Mondino de' Liuzzi at the University of Bologna, in which capacity she is said to have developed a new method of draining blood vessels and then refilling them with hardened dyes to make vessel identification and tracing easier and more accurate. She is said to have died at the age of 19 from a septic wound incurred in the line of her work. Some historians believe she was a figure invented by later authors.

Abella (fourteenth century)

According to Renatus Moreau's 1625 *Schola Salernitano de Valetudine*, Abella was a physician and lecturer at the Salerno School of Medicine. She wrote the now lost treatises *De atrabile* (On the Black Bile) and *De natura seminis humani* (On the Nature of Seminal Fluid), and was apparently, like Rebecca Guarna, interested in embryology.

Ameline (fourteenth century)

Ameline was a Parisian physician who was charged by the state with illegally practising medicine.

Adelmota of Carrara (fourteenth century)

According to the seventeenth-century writer Rhodius, Adelmota was an obstetrician and general physician who worked in Padua in the mid-fourteenth century and was married to James, the Prince of Carrara.

Dorotea Bucca/Bocchi (1360–1436)

Dorotea was the daughter of Giovanni di Bocchino Bocchi, a professor of medicine at the University of Bologna, and was herself a teacher at that institution from 1390 onwards. There is some debate as to whether she was a lecturer in medicine, or philosophy, or both.

Clarisse of Rotomago/Clarice of Rouen (early fourteenth century)

Clarisse was a French midwife who was arrested and excommunicated by the Prior of Sainte-Genevieve in 1312 for practising medicine.

Jeanne Converse (early fourteenth century)

Active in the early fourteenth century, Jeanne Converse was a French physician who was prosecuted for practising medicine without a licence, and subsequently excommunicated from the Catholic Church.

Maria Gallicia (early fourteenth century)

A Neapolitan surgeon specialising in gynaecological surgery, Gallicia received her licence in 1309, which restricted her to the performance of procedures related to the womb.

Mercuriade (fourteenth century)

Another product of the University of Salerno, Mercuriade was a physician and surgeon, and the author of the texts *De Febre Pestilenti* (Of Pestilential Fever), *De Curatio* (Of the Treatment of Wounds), and *De Ungentis* (Of Healing Salves).

Leonetta De Gorzano (fourteenth century)

Wife of Italian physician Giovanni di Gorzano, Leonetta is believed to have practised as a physician herself in Padua and Turin.

Sara of Saint-Gilles (fourteenth century)

A French doctor of Jewish descent, Sara of Saint-Gilles is known today from a contract signed on 28 August 1326 whereby she agreed to provide medical training for a Christian student named Salvet de Bourgneuf for a period of seven months.

Constanza/Constance Calenda (early fifteenth century)

Calenda was the daughter of the dean of medicine at the University of Salerno, where she is known to have passed a medical examination.

Subsequently, her father went on to the University of Naples, where Calenda perhaps obtained a doctor of medicine degree, which if true would have made her the first person in Europe to earn such a distinction.

Sara of Wurzburg (fifteenth century)

Women physicians from Germany were a rare enough thing in the Middle Ages, but Jewish German women physicians were rarer still. We know of Sara because she is recorded as having been charged ten florins annually to practise medicine because of her Jewish ancestry.

Chapter 3

Lady Mary Montagu and Europe's First Tool Against Smallpox

In the seventeenth century, smallpox ravaged Europe with a persistent ferocity beyond reckoning. At its height, it killed 400,000 Europeans a year, in a manner so painful and dehumanising that the modern mind can hardly encompass the scale of suffering. By the time vaccination had eradicated the disease in the late twentieth century, it had claimed upwards of 500 million lives, more than those lost in every war ever fought during the entire span of human history.

The story of Edward Jenner employing cowpox in 1798 to vaccinate against smallpox is justly one of modern science's most oft-told tales, but what is less often remembered is that the road for Jenner's success had been paved eighty years previously by a British woman who braved public ridicule to bring to Europe a practice of Ottoman origin: inoculation.

The woman was Lady Mary Wortley Montagu (1689–1762). The daughter of the Duke of Kingston upon Hull, she was born in the lap of unspeakable luxury. Her mother died when she was 3, and she lived with relatives until she rejoined her rakish father at the age of 9, where she had the opportunity to experience at first hand the rowdy world of British letters. Her father was a member of the Kit Cat Club, a group of nobles who gathered for the express purpose of getting very drunk and writing poems about which eligible British women they thought were the most attractive. Thrust into this world of sparkling if superficial wit, and hailed for her beauty and mind alike, she resolved to become the centre of learned attention by devoting herself to study.

Her father possessed a large library and placed no restrictions upon her access to it, and she employed it to learn those things her teachers had refused her: Latin, classical studies and philosophy. She turned author herself and wrote poems depicting the mad pace and loose morals of British high society.

She developed a theory of romance inspired by the divisions of the Catholic afterlife and introduced her friends to her novel system. There were marriages of Paradise, cemented on a firm base of passionate intellectual and physical love, those of Hell, filled with grotesque and fearsome husbands, and those of Limbo, where the money was good enough to provide comfort and the husband bland enough to not be an active hindrance. As it happened, Lady Mary set her sights on Paradise, nearly tumbled into Hell, and landed firmly in Limbo.

Beautiful and witty, Lady Mary had no shortage of suitors but decided ultimately on Edward Wortley Montagu, a wealthy businessman and energetic MP eleven years her senior, whose circle of acquaintances included some of London's greatest writers and satirists. He valued, or appeared to, her intellectual gifts, and soon the couple was secretly corresponding through a series of loyal intermediaries. In due course, Wortley entered into marriage talks with Lady Mary's father, but refused her father's terms as to how he was to dispose of his property in his will, and the negotiations broke down.

This was just as well from the point of view of Kingston (now marquess of Dorchester), as he had what was to his mind a superior match lined up with the fabulously named the Honourable Clotworthy Skeffington, a non-intellectual bore who made Lady Mary's blood run cold. Her father made her choice clear: marry Skeffington or be disinherited. She considered the matter, and opted against Hell; with her brother's help, she eloped with Wortley in 1712 while on the road to meet Skeffington. True to his word, Kingston cut off all contact and support, but Wortley had more than enough money to make up the loss.

What he did not have, it turned out, was a loving heart. Soon after their wedding night, he slid into a profound indifference towards Lady Mary, spending as much time as possible away from her and their first son. He made his position clear: he would support her but he would not be a regular feature of her life.

As such, Lady Mary Montagu took her diversion where she could, finding favour in the eyes of King George I and his son as a sparkling addition to Court. Her position as a universally envied Court favourite, however, ran to little longer than a year, as in 1715 she caught smallpox. She survived, but the disease left her face and body a pitted husk of its former self. 'Pitted and pitied', the saying went, and it was a long time before she could bring herself to venture outside without her face hidden beneath a silk veil.

Her life, however, took on new direction suddenly in 1717 when her husband was appointed ambassador to the Ottoman Empire for the purpose of brokering peace between the Ottomans and the Austrians. Here, in addition to writing some of Europe's first accounts of how women actually lived in Turkey, which would define a new genre of travel literature, she witnessed something truly remarkable: a ritual practised by the Turkish women that seemed to all but ensure immunity to smallpox.

Their practice was to lightly scratch the skin, apply some matter from the pock of a person who had one of smallpox's mildest forms, and to cover the whole with a walnut shell. The people so treated developed a mild pox that passed without leaving any scars, and carried lifelong immunity to all forms of smallpox, including the confluent variety that caused bleeding from the eyes and virtually guaranteed death.

Transfixed by the simplicity and efficacy of the Ottoman women's solution to a disease that had cut through Europe like an avenging angel, she ordered the process performed on her son. The procedure was a complete success, and Lady Mary knew at once news of it must be brought to England, if only the medical establishment there could look beyond its professional, racial and gender pride long enough to learn a new method from the traditional culture of a group of coloured, non-Christian, women.

Her homeland was, however, decidedly unreceptive to the notion of inoculation – using pox to cure pox sounded like irresponsible quackery to ears trained in the techniques of bleeding, purging and cold cures, and nobody was willing to take a chance on it. So, Lady Mary seized the initiative and convinced the physician who had travelled with her in Constantinople to perform the procedure on her daughter to prove its validity. This he did, accompanied by several learned English doctors. When the child, a child of the highest class, made a full recovery, word got around to the Royal family.

Smallpox had long been the scourge of royalty, upsetting carefully wrought lines of inheritance and the nations dependent upon them. King George soon gave his permission to have the process tested on six criminals who would be rewarded with their freedom for volunteering. These tests proving equally successful, British doctors began making inoculation their own, which is to say, very nearly ruining it.

Lady Mary watched in horror and rage as the simple, effective 'Scratch & Apply' process of the Turks warped in the hands of the British experts into a carnival of torture. Patients were purged (i.e., repeatedly and systematically induced to vomit) and bled before the procedure in order to 'prepare' them, and in place of the simple surface scratch the British medics used deep cuts which they stuffed with pock matter. Thinking that they had improved the process by introducing Western insights, they had in fact made it several orders more unnecessarily unpleasant, and even dangerous, for all concerned parties. Lady Mary took up her pen to write an anonymous letter calling her nation's doctors to account, but was scoffed at by a medical establishment that refused to believe its instincts inferior to those of a gaggle of non-Christian Turkish women.

In spite of British *improvements*, inoculation continued to rack up a growing wave of victories, precipitating a low-key mania for the process amongst the nobility, particularly after the king approved the inoculation of his own grandchildren. To those households who received the blessing of inoculation, Lady Mary was a hero, an indispensable presence at their children's procedures. But to many more, she was a pure villain – a woman promoting a procedure that infected perfectly healthy children with dreaded pox. They gathered in front of her house whenever she intended to attend an inoculation, throwing rotten fruit and eggs at her when she emerged, yelling insults at this woman who had become, in their mob-addled minds, the very personification of smallpox itself.

She, however, took the abuse in her stride. As long as a family needed her, she would go, and if she had raw egg in her hair, and needed to wear red to match the colour of a hurled tomato, well, that was a small price to keep others from suffering as she had.

Once inoculation had become established, doctors felt less inclined to seek Lady Mary's experience, and the remaining four decades of her life were spent trying to rein in her often-wayward offspring, composing philosophical and political letters, and rebuffing the advances of poet Alexander Pope only to fall in love with bisexual heart-throb Francesco Algarotti. She moved to France to live with him for three years, and remained in continental Europe for two decades, only returning to England upon hearing news of her husband's death. The woman who brought Great Britain its first weapon in the war against smallpox returned to her country at last in 1762, and died there seven months later.

Further Reading

The Speckled Monster: A Historical Tale of Battling Smallpox (2003) by Jennifer Lee Carrell is a work of history that reads like a grand work of literature. It is about Lady Mary but also about a parallel effort in the American colonies to introduce inoculation in Boston; both tales are gripping. Jo Willett's *The Pioneering Life of Mary Wortley Montagu* (2021) is also a great source. Lady Mary's sparkling form as a letter writer is well represented in a Penguin collection of her letters, and her Turkish Embassy letters are perennially in print. If you want to know more about her post-inoculation work and place in British literature, you will probably want to add either the Barry or Grundy biographies to your shelves.

Chapter 4

The Last of the Women Physicians

Dorothea Leporin Erxleben

Prior to the eighteenth century, the answer to the question, 'Who was allowed to practise medicine?' was relatively simple: just about anybody. While those who attended university were given a theory-based education in natural philosophy, it was left largely to the members of the community to carry out the day-to-day healing of the sick. A man possessing a doctorate might analyse a case and prescribe a regimen, but it was up to your barber to perform the actual surgery, your local apothecary to actually make the medicines he prescribed, and a whole network of experienced women to provide regular care.

In this world, the wife of a pastor was likely to have more practical experience of useful medical techniques than the most respected and betitled of university physicians, and was honoured by the community accordingly as someone who prescribed what worked rather than what ought to work. In the Age of Enlightenment, however, these old roles were rapidly changing. States were centralising, and countries like Prussia, where the maintenance of the army and robustness of the economy dominated government policy, began taking a serious interest in the haphazard practice of medicine throughout the land.

Sick people were not productive people, and so *professional standards* were necessary – approved university standards that clearly delineated who was allowed to practise medicine and who was not. Those standards ultimately worked to the overwhelming good of society, as they slowly ground out the superstition and quackery that run rampant in any decentralised medical system, but in the short term they had the effect of pushing a number of the nation's greatest practical medical practitioners out of medicine.

One woman, however, refused to be pushed. Dorothea Leporin (1715–1762) was the daughter of a Quedlinburg doctor who had made his name in sensibly avoiding the extremes of the medical profession's various fads, prescriptions and theories. As a child, she was constantly falling ill, one disease leading to the next in an almost seamless progression.

Weakened physically, the time in her bed gave her mind free range to roam where it would, inspired by the example of the polymath and proto-feminist Anna Maria van Schurman (1607–1678). She showed an early interest in science, which her father was only too happy to guide, and, as her body grew stronger, the passing interests of the sick bed became a central interest of her life as her father took his talented daughter under his wing and started teaching her the doctor's trade.

She was educated side by side with the most talented of her brothers (the other siblings were wisely allowed by their parents to go their own ways as individuals 'Not Suited to Learning'). In 1740 that brother, Christian Polycarp, was given leave by his regiment to carry out university studies in Halle, only to have that decision rescinded in the autumn as Frederick II needed all soldiers to report for duty in preparation for his invasion of Silesia. Christian left Halle but did not rejoin his regiment. Meanwhile, his sister took the unprecedented step of writing to Frederick II directly, asking for permission for her brother to continue his studies and also the king's leave for herself to attend the university to continue her medical education. Frederick, ever the archetypal Enlightenment monarch, approved both.

This *should* be the point in the story where brother and sister trot arm in arm to Halle to receive a thoroughly Prussian education, and so it would have been had Christian rejoined his regiment when he had been ordered to. By ducking that command, Christian had technically been put down in the books as a deserter, which was a crime most dire in a country of such military character as eighteenth-century Prussia. Sorting through the paperwork and counter-paperwork of his case consumed time and in that time, Dorothea Leporin met Johann Christian Erxleben, a local deacon who was entirely in tune with Dorothea's continuing her medical work but who also came with children from a previous marriage who needed tending.

They were married in 1742, and in 1744 Dorothea gave birth to the first of a string of children. The plans for her to attend university were dropped, but, as Erxleben later reflected, she did not feel it as a great loss at the time. To do the sort of medical work she wanted to do, no university degree was required, and the experience and knowledge she had gained at her father's side were equal to those of any university-educated practitioner. What good would an extra piece of paper possibly be to her patients?

All this time, however, she had been sitting on a manuscript, which her father had urged her to write but that she delayed publishing (whether out of modesty or a fresh author's genuine need to not release their work until everything is polished to impossible perfection), the *Gründliche*

Untersuchung der Ursachen, die das Weibliche Geschlecht vom Studiren abhalten (1742). It was, in the tradition of van Schurman, a call to self-study for women that tore through the traditional arguments against their education and substituted instead an impassioned belief that communities become better places when everybody is allowed to explore the full extent of their mental abilities. More than a possibility, it was a duty for each woman possessing the means to educate herself and so demonstrate the true universality of reason and understanding.

Erxleben's father died in 1747, and she inherited not only his practice, but his various intellectual feuds as well. In life he had clashed with a Dr Grasshoff, who came from a long-established family and therefore had first claim to any positions within the local medical hierarchy no matter what his worth as an actual doctor. Dr Leporin had called into question his use of prescriptions and, while Grasshoff could not move against Leporin directly, his backers *could* descend en masse to attack Leporin's daughter when she stood alone, without his protection.

They seized their opportunity in February 1753 when one of her patients died. Losing a patient in the eighteenth century was of course not uncommon, but the Grasshoff camp clutched the moment to accuse Erxleben of Quackery and demanded of the government that she be stripped of her rights to practise medicine. Without missing a beat, Erxleben remembered that she had in her pocket the king's permission to attend university. She duly enrolled and somehow managed to complete her dissertation by January 1754, less than a year after the attack on her reputation, and only eight months after the birth of her last child.

She attended her oral examinations on 6 May that same year, a cross-examination carried out entirely in Latin, and in the estimation of her examiners showed accuracy and knowledge such as few had ever demonstrated. Grasshoff's attack had backfired tremendously. In attempting what he thought would be an easy win against a lone deacon's wife, he had in fact motivated her to attain a degree equal to his own, with a speed and ease that clearly demonstrated the mean-spirited vacuity of his claims, and had gained with it full protection against any future attacks he and his well-established coterie might concoct.

As much of a triumph and personal vindication as the degree was for Dorothea Erxleben, it was to be the last of its kind. As with Laura Bassi, once one woman showed herself the equal of the system, that system swiftly moved to ensure that others would not be given similar opportunities. In fact, it would be a century and a half before another woman received a medical degree in Germany.

Dorothea's husband died in 1759, and Dorothea herself followed three years later after a swift illness. She had, by her words, argued for women's right and duty to educate themselves, and for a medical practice that utilised the experience of its best practitioners to provide moderate cures for illnesses rather than chasing every costly medical fad. And by her actions, in practising and in attaining her degree, she had shown the expertise that experienced community-based medical care was capable of, even as that system was giving way to the steady centralising professionalism of the modern era. She was the first of her kind and the last of her kind, and who can say what medicine might have been had the Enlightenment allowed itself to follow its best principles more than just the once.

Further Reading

Erxleben's life is readily available in multiple scholarly biographies and novelisations in the German language, and in particular I like Eva Brinkschulte's 2006 *Dorothea Christiana Erxleben: Weibliche Gelehrsamkeit und medizinische Profession seit dem 18. Jahrhundert* as not only a good guide to Erxleben but to the gradual shift in the medical profession generally in the eighteenth century.

Chapter 5

Midwife to a Nation

Madame du Coudray and the King's Commission to Professionalise Childbirth

Midwife. Few words in the history of western medicine can evoke sudden and unequivocal academic tribal sentiment as that single term. To one school of thinking, the rise of the professional doctor and surgeon class to supplant local midwifery was a necessary precondition for the development of modern medicine and the curtailing of the infant mortality rate. For others, the doctors' assumption of the midwives' role was a usurpation by a jealous and organised body who sought to use their standing and administrative power to muscle out a dedicated and deeply experienced group of competitors from their highly skilled livelihoods, a gendered strike against the growing organisation of women professionals.

Those two conceptions of the midwife, as the experienced front-line hero of childbirth and as the doddering unschooled rural ignoramus, grew in intensity over the eighteenth century, and in one country centred on one particular figure, a tireless woman who trekked across the country armed with a king's commission to teach the art of childbirth wherever she went. She was Angélique Marguerite Le Boursier du Coudray (*c.*1712–1794), inventor, businesswoman, lecturer and an unrivalled expert in the subtle art of delivering babies, and the subtler art of teaching that skill to thousands of largely illiterate countrywomen in a way they could understand and bring back to their native villages.

Many surgeons deeply respected her craft, and came to her classes to learn, but as the years wore on and her mission extended across the towns and villages of France, training a new generation of women to confidently handle difficult childbirths without the need to consult the local male doctors, a stiff resistance to du Coudray – and by extension to all practising midwives – set in that sought to slander her in print and deprive her of the opportunity to do the work she had been royally appointed to do.

Against a less resolute woman, these tactics might have worked, but du Coudray was a force, who knew her worth to the nation and would not sit idly by while usurpers and slanderers attempted to diminish the value of her mission. Where she got this indomitable will, we shall probably never know, as the details of her first three decades of life are all but entirely lost. She first appears in the historical record in 1740, when she registered as a licensed midwife in Paris after a traditional three-year apprenticeship with Anne Bairsin. This was a costly licence to obtain, and prospective applicants had not only to pay a fee but pass an exam before a panel of medical notables, present testimony by a member of the clergy as to their religious character, and withstand the questioning of all their known friends to determine their moral rectitude.

The level of personal and professional probing was deemed necessary because of the midwife's legal and moral authority in early eighteenth-century Europe. Her expertise was often sought in legal cases, and her word was taken as truth in judgments about pregnancy, virginity and paternity. She was trusted by the local community as a protector of women having children out of wedlock, by the Church with the responsibility of presenting children at christenings, and by the state in determining biological facts pertaining to women that had legal significance. This status was looked upon with jealousy by not a few male medical practitioners, who felt that women's virtual monopoly on child birthing was something suspicious grounded in a superstitious femininity that must be supplanted by modern theory and technologies. Out with the practised hands of the midwife, in with the technical precision of the obstetrical forceps, invented in the sixteenth century, but seeing its first wide use now in the early eighteenth. For some time, the surgeons of Paris simply refused to hold the exams that would allow the creation of new midwives, claiming that there were too many already, leaving the midwife community, with du Coudray as one of its leading voices, to find alternate venues for medical instruction, skilfully playing the rival jealousies of the doctors and surgeons off one another in an attempt to gain knowledge and certification.

Growing in authority as one of the leading midwives of Paris, du Coudray eventually rose to the station of head midwife at the Hotel Dieu, where women could go to deliver their babies regardless of ability to pay. Here, approximately 1,500 children were delivered in a year, and du Coudray's experience in handling every conceivable malpresentation and natal complication would prove crucial in the formation of her legendary classes of the 1760s through to the 1780s. She was doing well, but there must have been a hunger for something more, for when in 1751 an Auvergne noble advertised a desire to have a midwife come to his estates to teach the peasants there about the art of child delivery, du Coudray leapt at the opportunity, leaving behind her apprentice and practice to try something new and promising.

Over the next few years, du Coudray developed a teaching programme unique in the history of Europe: a hands-on course that stressed practice over theory and for which she developed a machine, a fabric mock-up of a mother's womb and the baby within, which allowed the peasant girls studying with her to practise each of the malpresentations that du Coudray had encountered over her years at the Hotel Dieu. Later, she added fluid-filled sponges throughout the machine that accurately mimicked different warning signs and regular discharges that a midwife must recognise and interpret, but to begin with the simple but accurate fabric mannequin allowed women to practise complex delivery techniques that they might otherwise have to wait years in the field to experience and come to grips with.

In an era where traditional village matrons held rapid delivery as the greatest goal, and encouraged the mother to hop up and down if the process seemed to be taking too long (with predictable results), du Coudray focused on how the midwife could, by feel alone, recognise different unique birth conditions, and develop best strategies for dealing with each so that she was rarely taken by surprise and never inclined to dangerously rush a delivery. Her students were enthusiastic, and glowing reports of her ability to take a few dozen village peasants and change them into confident and skilled analysts and delivery practitioners spread through France, helped along in 1759 by her publishing the *Abrégé de l'art des Accouchements*, an illustrated manual on childbirth that would go through several, ever more elaborately diagrammed, editions in the years to come.

The *Abrégé* treated the presentation of childbirth in a radically new way. Instead of illustrations that lingered dramatically on the naked body of the mother, du Coudray adopted colour-coded X-ray like images of the womb and child within, complete with illustrated hands to represent what the midwife ought to be doing in each case. This was a book written for her students, women who might be illiterate but still could use the illustrations as reminders of what to do in particular cases, while those who could read were treated to a medical text which forsook questionable theory and impenetrable jargon for practical advice in understandable terms.

Du Coudray's work came at an important time in French history, when demographic experts were warning of a coming population implosion fuelled by the scourge of rural infant mortality rates. The state, which ordinarily kept itself at a far remove from such issues, was suddenly intensely interested in the quality of child delivery in France. Too many babies were dying at birth, and too many of those that survived were disfigured or disabled by reckless delivery methods, and it was starting to tell on the bottom line of national productivity. Just as ministers were convincing themselves that something had to be done, du Coudray's book and courses were earning her national fame as *the* nation's expert on midwife instruction. A radical idea took shape in Paris, approved enthusiastically by the king – why not give this woman a royal commission to travel throughout France, teaching women village by village, and thereby exponentially multiplying her priceless knowledge on a national scale?

There was no precedent for such a commission, but seemingly desperate times called for new ideas, and du Coudray was duly given a royal *brevet*, a commission with the full weight of the Crown behind it, to go wherever she thought she could do the best work, and to collaborate with local governments to find potential midwife candidates and train them using her established methods. For the next two decades, from 1761 to 1783, du Coudray would do just that. District overseers lavishly competed with each other for the honour of a visit from the famous teacher and midwife, enthused by tales of wild success in locale after locale, of classrooms filled with 100 women turned in the course of three intense months into sophisticated experts in the art of complicated child delivery. Du Coudray drove herself hard, travelling the length and breadth of the country, sorting finances, organising teaching and living spaces, constructing and selling new teaching machines to be used by trained demonstrators once she left a locale, and building up a network of enthusiasts who would be her first line of defence against the increasingly shrill criticism being heaped upon her by a male medical establishment who saw nothing but threat in the growing legion of competent women practitioners.

She was not welcome everywhere. A few surgeons had taken all-out war against midwives as their life's cause, and where they reigned supreme, du Coudray was not allowed to even offer her class. The surgeons saw the often-brutal condition of rural childbirth, and decided the solution lay not in an organised and knowledgeable education of a new generation of midwives, but in the total elimination of women from the profession of child delivery. Women, so these surgeons wrote, lacked the mental capacity to understand the theory of medicine, and in focusing so closely upon one aspect of the body, were liable to critically miss important secondary circumstances that impacted upon childbirth. It was the eighteenth century, medicine was professionalising itself, and there was no room in it anymore for these women claiming some traditional competence.

The attacks on du Coudray became more virulent as her successes grew more conspicuous. The medical establishment used its power to keep her name out of official medical journals, and to promote rival childbirth manuals written by sanctioned male authors, even sending them to the towns where she was teaching to try and trick her students into buying them. They built and advertised birth demonstration machines to compete with her own and lobbied the government to end her mission, compelling her on numerous occasions to return to the capital, armed with reams of testimonials of the importance and success of her work, to forcefully re-establish and extend her authority.

By virtue of an indomitable will, in spite of the coordinated attacks of an entire profession, du Coudray held on to her role (and even began collecting a regular salary instead of a conditional stipend) and continued travelling and teaching into her early seventies before handing over her title and authority to the adoptive niece who had been her steady helper since the virtual beginning, Madame Coutanceau. Coutanceau, for her part, would go on to become the first woman to run a medical clinic in France, and continued du Coudray's mission of midwife instruction into the early nineteenth century. As for du Coudray herself, increasing weight and age forced her at last to retire from her relentless schedule in the early 1780s, and as France plunged into the French Revolution, her future was anything but secure. On one hand she was lauded as a patriot who brought knowledge to the dark superstitious corners of the nation, on the other she was under suspicion as a long-time employee of the now disgraced royal family.

Her pension, and her niece's fees for teaching midwifery, stopped being paid by the state – in spite of an official inquiry which showed the overwhelming impact of her work in the provinces. Testimonials and statistics poured in detailing the impact of her mission, the students trained who went on to train further generations in a radiating pulse that touched all corners of the land. But whatever information one government collected was lost to the next as Assembly succeeded Assembly and the Terror sank its claws into the national consciousness. Du Coudray and Coutanceau somehow kept themselves from starving, and even managed to keep Coutanceau's clinic open and running, but agents of the Terror increasingly had them under surveillance.

It was under these circumstances, reduced to near penury and living in fear, that Madame du Coudray breathed her last, probably as a result of the shock and stress of an interrogation at the hands of Jacobin agents attempting to establishing her 'patriotic' credentials. Her last moments are as much a mystery as her first decades, her legacy all but buried in the mad rush of a medical community attempting to fully professionalise itself. She was virtually lost in the medical record until historians recently, out of a renewed interest in the story of the interface between midwives and surgeons, painstakingly began piecing together the tale of European midwifery in the early Modern age. Her impact, they discovered, was vast, not only in the innovation of using demonstrative models to teach delivery methods, or in publishing a child delivery textbook that employed cutting edge publishing and illustrative techniques to show the most important aspects of the birthing process, but in the radiating waves of influence resulting from her insistence on teaching young and promising but uneducated rural women in ways that they could understand and pass along. The knowledge of one woman became the expertise of thousands, and the population of France thrived in the century to come under that expertise.

Further Reading

One scholar went above and beyond the call of historical duty to painstakingly assemble all of the existent letters by and to du Coudray in an attempt to recreate and document the complicated travels of Louis XV's revolutionary teacher. She is Nina Rattner Gelbart and I saw her work first in a compilation of essays about the history of midwifery (*The Art of Midwifery: Early Modern Midwives in Europe* (1993)), and in one of the footnotes she mentioned she was preparing a full-scale book on the topic of Madame du Coudray, to be titled *Delivering the Goods: The Midwife Mission of Mme du Coudray in eighteenth-century France*, at which point I instantly sought out the prospective book only to find that its title ended up being *The King's Midwife: A History and Mystery of Madame du Coudray* (1998), which disappointed me because I do love a good silly pun in the title of an academically rigorous work; however, the book itself is wonderful. Deeply researched with regard to both du Coudray's peregrinations and the history of the conflict between medical professionals and rural women practitioners, it lifts the veil on a bygone time to tell a story almost too heroic to be true.

Chapter 6

Brief Portraits

Women Physicians of the Early Modern Era

Grace Sherrington Mildmay (~1552–1620)

A member of the English nobility, Grace Sherrington was taught medicine by her governess, Mistress Hamblyn. In the ensuing years, she collected a large collection of medical volumes and papers, and made herself an expert on *materia medica*. From her base at Apethorpe Palace in Northamptonshire, she practised medicine throughout the neighbourhood, mixing her own cures in 10-gallon vats. The autobiography she wrote, which was not published until 1911, ranks among the earliest penned by an English woman.

Olivia Sabuco Banera D'Alcaraz (1562–1588)

Sabuco was the Spanish author of the 1587 treatise *Nueva Filosofia de la Naturaleza del Hombre* (*New Philosophy of Human Nature*) which is an early document in the history of holistic medicine. She believed that emotions were a critical component of health, and played a role in the balance of the body's humours which had to be taken into consideration when devising new cures.

Louise Bourgeois Boursier (1563–1636)

The most famous of French historical midwives before the arrival of Coudray, Bourgeois first took up midwifery when the French religious civil war compelled her to flee her home with her children and find paying employment. The surgeon Ambroise Paré was an acquaintance of the family, and for five years she observed him at work. In 1593, she joined the Guild of Midwives, and in 1598 passed the examinations to receive her official registration. By 1601, she had become the Royal Midwife to Henry IV, in which capacity she oversaw the birth of Louis XIII as well as

Marie de Medici's subsequent five children. In 1609/10 she published her first book on obstetric theory, *Various Observations on the Sterility*, which was expanded in multiple subsequent editions, and included descriptions of problem cases, abortion, mother and child aftercare, and a method for induced labour invented by Bourgeois.

Jane Sharp (*c.*1641–1671)

We know virtually nothing of Jane Sharp's life outside of her authorship of England's first guide to midwifery penned by a woman, *The Midwives Book, or, the Whole Art of Midwifery Discovered.* It was an influential book for many reasons – it was addressed not only to practising midwives but to men and women who wanted to learn more about anatomy and the processes of child conception, growth and birth. It was written in the vernacular rather than in Latin, and featured a minimum of technical terminology. And, of course, it was written by a woman who had served as a midwife for thirty years at the point of the book's first publication, and thus had first-hand experience of a process that many male authors of midwifery guide books only knew theoretically.

Madeleine-Francoise Calais (~1713-?)

Claimed by Paul-Martin Bondois as the First Woman Dentist in France, Calais studied with the dentist Gerandly of Paris from 1732 to 1735, then served as his assistant from 1735 to 1740. In 1740, she applied for a licence from the Surgical Society of Paris, which referred the issue all the way up to the king's royal surgeon before deciding that, yes, her petition for a licence would be allowed, making her the first fully licensed woman dentist in the country.

Regina Josepha (née Henning) von Siebold (1771–1849)

Josepha von Siebold was the first woman to earn a doctorate in obstetrics from a German University. After her father died when she was young, she was placed in the care of a family friend whom she married when she was 15 years of age. After his death, she remarried, this time the doctor in whose care she had been placed when she fell ill. This was not an era that was big on resisting the urge to take advantage of power dynamics. In any case, she was soon an assistant in her husband's medical practice and eventually wanted to strike out on her own as an obstetrician, attending classes at the University of Wurzburg from behind a curtain. She petitioned and received permission from the Grand Duke of Hesse-Darmstadt to take the final exams at the university, which she passed without difficulty in 1807, followed by a doctorate from the University of Giessen in 1815. She and her daughter (see below) managed a charity clinic for a number of years.

Charlotte Marianne Heidenreich von Siebold (1788–1859)

The daughter of Josepha von Siebold from her first marriage, Charlotte was adopted by Damian von Siebold, and followed in her mother's footsteps, earning a degree in obstetrics from the University of Giessen in 1817, two years after her mother earned her historic doctorate from the same institution. In 1819, she was an assistant at the birth of the future Queen Victoria, and a few months later assisted at that of Victoria's future husband, Prince Albert.

Margaret Ann Bulkley/James Miranda Stuart Barry (1795–1865)

The lengths that Margaret Bulkley had to go to in order to practise medicine are a sign of how far the profession of woman physician had fallen since its pre-modern Italian heyday. Born in Cork, Ireland, she was originally educated to become a tutor, but failing to find a suitable position, she and her family hatched the plan of creating James Barry, a male identity that would allow her to attend medical school in England, beginning in 1809. She received her MD in 1812, and in 1813 passed the Royal College of Surgeons of England examinations, taking up a post with the army that year. For the next four and a half decades, until her retirement in 1859, Margaret/James rose through the medical ranks in the army, serving in positions all across the empire, without being detected as a woman. Her secret was only revealed at last in 1865 when her corpse was being laid out for her funeral.

Marchesa Buttelini (eighteenth century)

Like Lady Mary Montagu, Marchesa Buttelini was an early advocate of smallpox inoculation, and performed that procedure in Rome with the approval of Pope Benedict XIV.

Zaffira Peretti (eighteenth century)

Peretti taught at the University of Ferrara until approximately 1780, when she moved to Ancona to oversee a midwife training school there. She subsequently received a degree from the University of Bologna somewhere around the year 1800.

Joanna Stephens (eighteenth century)

Stephens is known to us today as the inventor of a 'lithontriptic', or oral cure for bladder stones. By the eighteenth century, surgery was the preferred means of removing bladder stones but it was, to put it mildly, not a pleasant process to undergo. Stephens revived the ancient practice of creating a mixture that could be taken orally or injected into the bladder. Her concoction was remarked on by David Hartley in 1738 as seemingly remarkably effective. He proposed to gather £5,000 and offer it to Stephens if she would produce her formula for the mixture and agree to its being tested on four individuals to ascertain its effectiveness empirically. She agreed, the mixture was administered, and the four patients recovered, entitling Stephens to the then-astronomical sum of £5,000. (Her recipe, in case you are curious, relied primarily on egg shells, snails, honey and soap. It was later determined that the high lime content of the mixture was responsible for its efficacy.)

Chapter 7

Lavinia Waterhouse

Gold Rush Physician, Frontier Suffragette

Lavinia Waterhouse (1809–1890) lived at the intersection of a tangle of ideas that, to the twenty-first-century mind, have no business being together. She was a physician – practising in the midst of California's Gold Rush – who was also a Spiritualist, who was also a poet and artist, who was also a leading suffragist, who was also a businesswoman (at least during the rare intervals when Sacramento managed to not be critically flooded or on fire). That combination of hard-nosed practicality and artistic whimsy, baffling to us, formed a cohesive and sensible whole in the nineteenth century, each part reinforcing the others in subtle ways that tended not to survive the technocratic crush of the modern age.

Lavinia Gertrude Goodyear was born in 1809 in New York, and of the first sixteen years of her life we know absolutely nothing. It was not until 1825, when both her parents died, that Lavinia stepped into history. Losing both parents simultaneously was a *very* nineteenth-century sort of occurrence that kicked off a string of *supremely very* nineteenth-century biographical happenings. She was married at the age of 21 to Charles Waterhouse, a tuberculosis-ridden man with whom she had thirteen children of whom only *three* survived. Three.

That alone goes far to explain how all of Lavinia Waterhouse's complicated interests hung together. When you have to bury ten children, Spiritualism, or the belief that one can communicate with the dead, takes on an aching plausibility, aided by the fact that the Spiritualists, unusual amidst the religious landscape of the long nineteenth century, practised total gender equality, a cause that would form a major part of Waterhouse's public existence.

That would be in the future, but to return to the cavalcade of misery, Waterhouse and her husband decided to move out West in 1852, lured by the promise of California's clean air and water that were reputed to magically cure all ailments. Disease, it was advertised, was impossible in the new state, so bring the children! The family set out, hoping that the change would cure Charles of his tuberculosis. As it happened, he died in 1856, just three years after finally reaching Sacramento, leaving Lavinia to raise their children by herself in a frontier town that alternately flooded or caught fire with amazing regularity.

She had survived a full year of covered-wagon travel west, the death of ten children, and her own husband's sad and inevitable end. The only options were to marry again, to give up and head back east, or to go into business for herself. She chose the latter, advertising as a physician and midwife specialising in the application of the Water Cure.

Becoming a doctor with minimal formal training was a relatively common practice at the time. The most 'formally educated' of male doctors had typically only two years of actual study, followed by a brief apprenticeship, followed by a slap on the back and the best of wishes to not kill too many patients. Regulation in the civilised East was sporadic, and in the loose-and-fast West was virtually non-existent. So, to up and declare one's self a practising physician was not, in that locale, madly eccentric, nor was the choice to specialise in the Water Cure.

The Water Cure, which attempted to cure patients of disease through an interminable and rigorous schedule of bathing and water consumption, was one of the few areas of medical practice where women could operate freely. The science behind it was virtually non-existent, but then again, so was the science behind most things that professional male doctors employed at the frontier. But the Water Cure practitioners had something going for them that others did not: a commitment to women's public health that did not balk before Victorian prudery.

Waterhouse made her office a centre where women could come to be honestly informed about the state of their body, and taught about their potential diseases and health risks without the condescension and paternal obfuscation that they tended to receive from their more traditional doctors. In addition, as a midwife, Waterhouse never lost a single mother, a record not even approached by pre-sterilisation hospitals where doctors would not even bother to rinse their hands between cases, dragging diseases from patient to patient with appalling disregard for the resulting mortality rates.

Through her practice as a physician and her interest in Spiritualism, Waterhouse was brought deeper into the public gender issues of her day, and it was therefore inevitable that she would sooner or later involve herself in the women's suffrage movement. Beginning around 1870, she started writing letters to the Sacramento papers arguing for voting and economic rights, and composing pro-suffrage poetry for the leading feminist papers of the time – while also painting pictures based on women's rights themes.

And all the while, she maintained her practice through the most tumultuous years of Sacramento's history. Her place of business was destroyed on one or two occasions by natural disaster, and survived the crazed and haphazard building spree that elevated the entire downtown by 18 feet to avoid future destruction – whole buildings being hand-cranked upwards by teams of labourers while new earth and foundation was filled in beneath. The woman who had been thrown on to her own devices by disease and transplantation was, it turned out, unbreakable. Her reputation for providing clean and efficient medical service and honest, unvarnished advice during a time of unchecked frontier charlatanry kept the customers coming, even when there was no building for them to come to.

Now, some of you might be raising a sceptical eye about Lavinia Waterhouse being included in a collection of Women in Science. 'Water curing? That's not medicine, that's just frontier hornswoggling! What next, some stripe of mesmerist, perhaps?! Harrumph.' I hear and understand your harrumph, but Waterhouse is a crucial figure to know and understand for so many reasons. She was one of the front-line practitioners on the hazy cusp of modern medicine, trying to do as much good as she could within the permitted social confines, like thousands of others stumbling about the mid-nineteenth century trying to determine which way science would definitively break.

She made women's health a public issue, and supported its progress by the fruit of her own business acumen, working just as hard at treating patients individually as she did at raising public awareness of women's institutionally enforced self-ignorance. She embodies a cluster of beliefs and practices born of tragedy and oppression, held together by the need for community and some ultimate permanence, and that is something also good to keep in mind whenever we moderns scoffingly slide into 'Victorians Were Dumb, Effete and Gullible' mode. Her story illuminates her time.

She married again, perhaps to one of Sacramento's most notorious frivolous lawsuit litigants ever. Or perhaps the man just had the same name. She did not keep him around long enough for anything more than his name to enter into the permanent record. Her daughter, who had been her constant companion during the lean, hard, early years, died in childbirth at the hands of a traditional doctor, another notch of misery on the severely hacked rod of Waterhouse's life. She saw women's suffrage fail when it was brought to vote in 1879, and retired soon after that, living her remaining eleven years in relative obscurity in Monterey County, where she had acquired numerous tracts of land.

Upon her death in 1890, she bequeathed all her Pacific Grove property to the building of a retirement home for elderly women, a final act of consideration capping a life of hard scrabble frontier empathy and devotion.

Further Reading

You will not be surprised that there is not much written about Lavinia Waterhouse. I came across her almost entirely by accident in Cheryl Anne Stapp's *Disaster and Triumph: Sacramento Women, Gold Rush Through Civil War*. It is an interesting book generally, which works hard to track down the decaying threads of these women's lives before they disappear forever. If it were not for this volume, we would have nothing about her except a tombstone and a girl's diary buried in the Sacramento archives, so grab one if you are at all curious about how women navigated the odd, paradoxical world of the early West.

Chapter 8

Founder's Curse

The Hard Rise and Long Fall of Elizabeth Blackwell, the First English Woman MD

The long life of Elizabeth Blackwell (1818–1910), the world's first English woman to earn a medical degree, can be divided into two roughly equal parts: four decades of being attentively reviled, followed by four decades of being respectfully ignored, and it is hard to say which was worse.

Her trailblazing years saw her in constant poverty, attempting to do what no woman in the modern age had yet done, all while suffering the loss of an eye and under intensely negative public scrutiny. But then, finally having climbed the mountain, sure of her pre-eminence in the newly emerged field of women doctors, she found herself quickly eclipsed, overrun by a new wave of practitioners whom her struggles had made possible, but who did not feel themselves bound to the Blackwell Model which had gone from revolutionary to old-fashioned in the course of a bit less than two decades.

The Blackwell siblings, of whom Elizabeth was the third of nine, were all a remarkable lot, and included Anna, who sampled seemingly every health and communal living fad of the nineteenth century, Henry, who married suffragette Lucy Stone and became a noted suffragist himself, and Emily, whose skills as a surgeon and cool head as the director of the Blackwells' Infirmary for Indigent Women and Children were both sources of pride and jealousy to her older, more famous, sister.

Their parents were both religious non-conformists of impeccable devoutness but possessed of a corresponding streak of doctrinal intolerance that would become a hallmark of Elizabeth's later career. Their father made and lost the family fortune in the slavery-dependent sugar business, in spite of being an avid abolitionist. From this mixture of high principle, deep combative faith and irreconcilable guilt came Elizabeth Blackwell. It gifted her an inflexibility in the face of adversity which would hold her in good stead through the frustrations of her early career, just as it gave her a moral rigidness that turned much of the latter half of her career towards a series of high-minded but ultimately fruitless and reactionary crusades.

When Elizabeth was 11 her family moved from England to America after a fire wiped out her father's sugar business. Hoping to re-establish themselves in the New World, the family moved to New York and settled into what would become decades of steady and demoralising financial decline. In 1838, Blackwell's father died suddenly, leaving behind a pile of debt and no clear path to paying it off. The professional options for a respectable, newly widowed woman were few – there was teaching, running a boarding house, and that was more or less the extent of it. The Blackwells, always a family devoted to education, decided to open a school and it was here that Elizabeth Blackwell realised that, fundamentally, she did not enjoy teaching.

But money was scarce, and options few, so for the next few years Elizabeth moved from appointment to appointment, scratching together what income she could as a classroom and private teacher in various communities throughout the South. The work was infuriating and unfulfilling as, day by day, Elizabeth had to choke back her rage at the casual cruelty of the slave owners around her and find a way to still be an effective teacher in towns that did not hold her knowledge in any regard.

Meanwhile, the germ of an idea had been placed in her head while attending the bedside of a dying friend. That friend had expressed frustration at always having to avail herself of the medical services of men. Why were there no women practising medicine to whom a woman could turn? Elizabeth considered the matter. She knew herself to be decidedly averse to being in the vicinity of an ailing body, and everybody she asked told her that it was madness to even consider becoming a doctor. Nobody would take a woman as an apprentice, and even if they did, no medical school would take a woman as a student, and even if they did, no hospital would allow a woman to establish a residency in order to gather experience, and even if they did, no patient would possibly want a woman as a doctor. Any attempt to become a doctor would be an expensive and depressing exercise in futility.

Blackwell being Blackwell, however, the more people protested as to the impossibility of her plan, the more she felt the necessity of seeing it through. To earn money and gain experience, she took teaching jobs that allowed her to study in her spare time with local doctors who, pushing tradition to the side, agreed to instruct her in medicine while she hunted for a medical college that might be persuaded into accepting her.

Beginning in 1845, she started acquiring direct experience of the medical profession and found that, though she was not as disgusted by disease and injury as she had worried, she was also growing a good deal more sceptical about the effectiveness of most contemporary medical cures and practices. As with so much in Blackwell's life, this exposure to the confused practices of nineteenth-century medicine had lasting effects both good and ill: it taught her not to invasively over-treat illness when simple rest and nutrition might suffice, but it also gave her an over-confidence in expressing scepticism about the utility of surgery, vaccinations and medical research that would ultimately damage the solidity of her medical reputation.

That was all far in the future, however, when, in 1847, she miraculously received word from Geneva Medical College that her application for admission had been forwarded to the student body and they had unanimously voted to let her join. Much has been made of the background to this historical acceptance – how the administration of the college only considered the application out of deference to a famous doctor who championed Blackwell's cause, and believed that, in passing it to the students, they were effectively ensuring her rejection, and how the students, taking the application as a joke, voted to accept her as part of the spirit of the presumed joke. However muddled the manner of her acceptance, there is no doubt that, once arrived, she made a reputation for herself as a competent and diligent learner, and the students soon demonstrated their entirely authentic regard for her when they voted to allow her to attend the anatomy sections that the college wanted to ban her from.

In the mid-nineteenth century, medical school was nowhere near the ordeal in perseverance it is today. You took classes for half the year over the course of two years and, at the end, you got your degree. Though an improvement over the old apprentice system, by which basically anybody could declare themselves a doctor, the knowledge one received by the end of those two years was not remotely comprehensive, and most of the actual learning of the doctoring trade was expected to be picked up out in the field in private practice or a hospital. Blackwell graduated in 1849, becoming the first woman in history to hold a modern medical degree.

The event attracted a fair amount of media attention, and a withering amount of professional commentary as medical journals outdid themselves in outrage over the slippery slope to which Geneva had just committed the entire profession. The College rapidly realised the depths of the scorn they had called down on their heads and resolved to close out all women candidates in the future.

But the damage had been done. Blackwell was through, and now had to shoulder the awesome responsibility of demonstrating to the world that a woman doctor could succeed. She realised that one missed diagnosis, one patient casualty, was all it would take for the establishment to, with a resounding Told You So, shut down the idea of women doctors forever. She needed more training, and the best place in the world for that was Paris, where she eventually took a job at La Maternité as essentially a midwife-in-training, in spite of her unique and infamous degree.

It was a step down in terms of prestige, but a great advance in terms of experience, and provided some of the most satisfying moments of Blackwell's career until one day, while treating a patient with the eye disease *ophthalmia neonatorum*, some disease-carrying fluid accidentally spurted into her own eye. Degeneration of the optical tissue followed, and with it encroaching blindness until the only solution was the removal of the infected eye. Whatever dreams she had of showing the world what a woman surgeon could do were over, as her remaining eye, though partially recovered, did not give her anywhere near the clarity required for that profession. For the rest of her life, she had to deal with the constant irritation of a series of variously well-constructed false eyes, and even the act of reading for prolonged periods became a torment.

By 1851, Blackwell had returned to the United States and established herself in practice in New York under the long shadow of Madame Restell. Restell had made her name and wealth as a skilful practitioner of abortions, and her name was as reviled as her services were sought. When the American public imagined a Woman Doctor in the mid-nineteenth century, it was Madame Restell who came to mind, and so when Blackwell set up her practice, she was widely believed to be little more than an abortion doctor hiding behind a medical degree. Paying patients were pitifully few in these hard years, and consisted almost entirely of members of the Quaker community who had always supported her career.

In 1853, frustrated with her foundering private practice, Blackwell struck out in a new direction, establishing a medical dispensary that offered services for New York's teeming masses of poor families. She was aided in this venture by a dynamic newcomer from Poland, Dr Marie Zakrzewska, whose innate genius for medicine was equalled only by her energy and ingenuity as a fundraiser. Together they reached out to the community to fund a larger dispensary which they launched in 1857 as the New York Infirmary for Indigent Women and Children.

This was a landmark moment in the history of medicine, as it gave women who had managed to obtain a medical degree a sorely needed place to gain practical experience. The Infirmary was staffed entirely by women, led by Blackwell's younger sister Emily, who was herself the third woman in United States history to obtain a medical degree and had a sparkling reputation for surgical skill. Together, Elizabeth, Marie and Emily made the Infirmary a running success which treated thousands of patients over the next decades and which survives to this day as the Lower Manhattan Hospital.

During the carnage of the Civil War, Blackwell attempted to organise medical aid to the US army through the founding of the Women's Central Relief Association, but in spite of her degree and first-hand experience running the Infirmary, the army gave the job of overseeing nurse training and distribution to Dorothy Dix, a schoolteacher with no formal medical training. Blackwell worked under her, overseeing the application process, anonymous but energetic in seeing that only the best and most dedicated volunteers entered the nursing service.

Cut off from a leadership role during the war, Blackwell's post-war years brought her one more definitive triumph as, again in combination with her sister Emily, she established the Women's Medical College. Most colleges still actively opposed women applicants, while the few institutions taking women were, by every observable metric, of decidedly second rate. Emily and Elizabeth decided that what was needed now was a women's college featuring first-tier professors and facilities where women could actually receive an education equal in quality and accessibility to that of men. One of the first students of the college was, in fact, Sophia Jex-Blake, who would go on to play a major part in the effort to open the British medical system to women.

Emily chaired the obstetrics department and Elizabeth that of hygiene and so, twenty-three years after first deciding to attempt for a medical degree, Elizabeth Blackwell found herself not only a doctor, but the founder of a hospital and a college, and the chair of a medical department. She did not know it, but this was the summit of her career, and it left her unsatisfied.

Always ready with a new grand plan, within a year Blackwell left the college she had founded and struck out for England to attempt to do for her native country what she had done for her adopted one. Emily stayed behind and, for the next four decades, ran the hospital and maintained her presence at the college, blossoming once out from under the shadow of her more famous sister.

Elizabeth, meanwhile, found that, though she was celebrated in England for her accomplishments, the cause of women in medicine was already well underway. Elizabeth Garrett Anderson, the first woman to earn a medical degree in England, led a Slow And Steady approach to convince the medical establishment of the reliability of women practitioners, while Sophia Jex-Blake organised a fiery circle of medical students who used litigation and dramatic appeals to the public to shame universities into accepting women students. Though temperamentally closer to Anderson than Jex-Blake, Blackwell soon found that she did not really fit in anywhere, and turned away from practising medicine to a new career as a social reformer.

This career met with decidedly mixed results. She had come to the conclusion that sex, while good in and of itself in the proper context, was being engaged in to such an outlandish degree that it was threatening the very bonds of society. She said, on the basis of no evidence in particular, that the more sex one had, the more one's health would suffer, and that the effect was even more pronounced for sex between members of different races. When England legislated, in the midst of an outbreak of syphilis, that prostitutes should be registered and their health regularly screened, Blackwell went on the offensive to repeal the bill and to educate the country away from the practice of prostitution altogether.

Meanwhile, she also spoke out as a strident critic of vivisection in medical research, of vaccinations, of the importance of surgery, and of Louis Pasteur's germ theory. She lambasted the century's greatest woman medical researcher, Mary Putnam Jacobi, for her attempts to use research to find the causes of disease, and took public exception to the frequency with which Elizabeth Anderson operated on her patients. To Blackwell's religiously inclined mind, the root cause of most sickness was a mixture of unclean conditions and moral laxity – if only people were more moral, and had more rest and better food, they would not succumb to illness. It was a view absolutely at odds with the amoral operators of germ theory or the detailed laboratory work of cellular biology, and it decisively isolated Blackwell from the living pulse of medical progress.

Alone in her beliefs, most of her friends long dead, and largely unheeded by a generation of women doctors whose lives were made possible by her impossible dreams and sacrifices, Elizabeth Blackwell spent her last years in the company of Kitty Barry, a woman she had adopted in 1856 as a girl of 7 with the expectation that she would be Blackwell's personal aide and helper for the rest of her life, and who was forbidden to marry or even entertain a suitor for as long as Blackwell was alive. She wrote books about her social morality theories, each of which sold fewer copies than the last, and an autobiography that virtually nobody read, and when she died at last in 1910, she was remembered as she was three-quarters of a century before – a daring innovator who pushed past poverty, injury and infamy to establish women in the medical field against titanic opposition, who gave the women who dared follow her a place to learn and a place to practise their new skills, and a complicated example to follow.

Further Reading

A new biography of Blackwell comes out every three decades or so, the easiest to find and most recent being Julia Boyd's *The Excellent Doctor Blackwell: The Life of the First Woman Physician* (2005) which is a great resource for balancing out Blackwell's personal drama (including the complicated combination of jealousy and pride wrapped up in her relationships with her siblings), her professional life, and her intricate relationship with the early women's rights movement (which we did not have space to go into here, but suffice to say, she was *against* it).

A bit harder to find, but worth the finding, are Ellen S. More's books on the history of women in modern medicine: *Restoring the Balance* (1999) and *Women Physicians and the Culture of Medicine* (2008). I also really like *'Send Us a Lady Physician': Women Doctors in America: 1835–1920* (1985), edited by Ruth J. Abram, as a collection of great essays, biographies and rare photos of nineteenth-century women doctors.

Chapter 9

Though the Profession Be Against You

Dr Elizabeth Garrett Anderson and the Battle for Medical Women

There are cases where the towering homogeneity of Victorian culture is exaggerated. The era of Prince Albert and Lord Palmerston was, after all, also the age of George Eliot, Charles Darwin and Karl Marx. Beneath the deceptive appearance of total societal conformity were swirling currents of dissent and radicalism that would shape the twentieth century once the Great War decisively threw Europe's staid self-confidence for a loop.

However, there are pockets of history where Victorianism's reputation for ramrod inflexibility and rank injustice are well-earned, and the story of medical women in the nineteenth century is among the most frustrating tales of that magnificently aggravating era. I am hard-pressed to think of an entire profession acting with such regular hypocrisy and calculated unity to shamefully hinder its own best interests in the name of social convention and popular prejudice as did the British medical community of the nineteenth century when presented with the desire of women to become practising doctors.

The pioneers in that movement suffered every imaginable indignity in their quest to learn and to work, a trial by fire that produced a vanguard of iron-willed practitioners who within decades summoned educational institutions, clinical associations and key legislation from the blank ether. That vanguard included the first British woman doctor, Elizabeth Blackwell, the founder of the London School of Medicine for Women, Sophia Jex-Blake, and the doctor, instructor, surgeon, organiser and administrator from whom all the movement's great projects ultimately stemmed: Elizabeth Garrett Anderson (1836–1917).

No step of her path was easy. Where a man's road to medical practice was smoothed by institutional regularity and strengthened by organisational membership, Garrett was compelled to act constantly in the shadows, snatching bits of learning and experience where she could, trying not to draw attention to herself lest her surreptitious learning sources be taken away. For a decade, she lived in the spaces of official doubt created by charter loopholes and bureaucratic disorganisation, achieving significant personal milestones only to see them closed behind her as institutions, horrified by what she had managed to accomplish, begrudgingly stole away the opportunities for future students to achieve even her hard-fought sliver of success.

For her first twenty-four years, Garrett's story was that of most daughters raised by tolerant, wealthy and liberal-leaning fathers of the Victorian age. She had been given an education better than most, including studies in Latin, French and German, and was regularly included in her father's discussions about European politics, which lessons she attempted to then pass on to her many younger siblings. She was smart and politically aware, but heading into her early twenties, had no direction for her energies and talents until her path chanced to fall across those of two of England's most remarkable women: Dr Elizabeth Blackwell, who had broken all convention when she earned a medical degree in the United States, and Emily Davies, who devoted herself to championing promising young women in their efforts to break into the professions.

Blackwell inspired Garrett, and Davies relentlessly pushed her to act on that inspiration, to find a way to stay in England and force its institutions to recognise her as a practising doctor. When her father heard of her plan, he was resistant at first but came around in quick order, and was her lifelong ally in the cause of advancing women's medical education. Her mother, on the other hand, locked herself away in her room, insisting that she was on the verge of dying of grief because of Garrett's decision. Family members flooded Garrett with letters begging her to put an end to her plans before her stubbornness killed her poor mother.

She did not end her plans, however, and her mother, you will be no doubt surprised to hear, did not expire of grief. Since all formal educational institutions were closed to her, she decided to gain some experience and test her resolve by volunteering as a surgical nurse for six months as a preliminary step. This was in 1860, and Lister's famous experiment using carbolic acid in surgery was five full years away, meaning that Garrett was to experience the full horror of pre-modern surgery. Doctors went from dissection theatre to the operating hall failing to wash their hands in between, and patients died at startling rates from infections even after minor surgeries. Tending those infections and observing those surgeries was Garrett's job, and it was taking the medical profession by the grizzliest end.

Her hospital had a medical school which of course refused her admittance but by virtue of her dedication and faultless record, she developed personal relationships with the doctors that opened subtle doors here and there. She was allowed into the dissecting rooms and given private lessons in *materia medica* and Greek by some of the profession's more luminous names. She was even allowed to attend some of the foundational chemistry lectures until one day when the professor asked a question and none of the male students knew the answer.

Garrett knew, and made the fatal mistake of raising her hand and giving the correct response. This was considered an outrage by the students and they circulated a petition to bar her from every aspect of the college, and to rescind every minor privilege she had clawed from the administration, an act of cowardly and selfish spite that is baffling still for its sheer smallness of spirit. Their motion carried, and Garrett was cut off from all avenues of official instruction.

Or very nearly. Through an oversight in its charter, the Society of Apothecaries had no clause that forbade women from receiving their medical credential. If she could find an apothecary to apprentice to, and pass the examination, there was legally nothing they could do to stop her from receiving their licence to practise medicine. She found a doctor willing to take her on, studied every waking hour to cram in all the Greek and Latin and chemistry and biology that she had missed in her youth, and after three years, in 1865, she passed the Society's exam with the highest score. She was to be a doctor after all.

In horror, the Society of Apothecaries closed its loophole after her victory. There remained no institutions that gave qualifying medical examinations in Britain, meaning that women had to take their exams in other countries to have any sort of certification at all, which would have been *something* were it not for the fact that the British medical community refused to recognise foreign certifications as legitimate. By closing off the last domestic institution that offered certification and refusing to admit the legitimacy of foreign certifications, England had effectively walled itself off completely from the possibility that women might contribute to its medical life.

But Elizabeth Garrett had slipped through before the final gate had swung shut, and she was determined to make her unique position count for as much as possible. She needed to show the country that a woman could be an effective doctor, *and* that many patients benefited tangibly from having the option of a woman doctor available to them. In 1866, she was a founding figure for St Mary's Dispensary for Women and Children, an institution staffed entirely by women. Garrett was the central force there, being the only certified doctor on staff, but she gathered around herself a crew of foreign-accredited women and aspiring students and the dispensary thrived. Women packed the waiting room, attracted by the reputation for excellent care and the chance to finally see a woman doctor who might actually *tell* them things instead of patronising them with Victorian obfuscations. Her dispensary proved that women benefited from access to women doctors, *and* proved that women doctors were efficient and capable of even the most complicated of surgical practices.

To bolster her credentials, Garrett went to Paris in 1870, took the medical examination there, *in French*, and overwhelmingly passed, adding another feather to the cap of the British women's medical movement, and increasing the prestige of her private practice, though of course doing nothing for her officially in the British medical community. When a restructuring of the British educational system was carried out that same year, it allowed women to stand for positions on school boards, and Garrett put her hat definitively in the ring, giving speeches to her constituency and winning the election in a landslide, earning 47,848 votes while her nearest competitor only pulled 13,494. Her chief strategist for that election was James Anderson, a steamship company owner who was intoxicated by her talent and drive and duly fell in love with her.

The two married in 1871 with the explicit understanding that Garrett would continue with her work. Anderson supported her efforts completely, even as their mad joint work schedule invited outside comment. Successfully established as a private doctor, with international and domestic certification, and a founding figure of an outrageously successful experimental hospital, Garrett had by no means expended her bag of tricks. She realised that membership in the British Medical Association would represent a massive advance for women doctors, so she obtained membership quietly through one of its more remote branches in 1873, remaining unobtrusively on the books for two years before arriving at meetings in London. Unable to deny her entrance, the Association nevertheless immediately moved that a statute be put on the books denying all future women applicants admission to the society.

Garrett, during the debates, rose and gave one of the great speeches of nineteenth-century feminism, laying out all that had been done already by women doctors, demonstrating that their numbers would only grow, and outlining how refusing all communication with this growing crop of practitioners was a deep betrayal of the basic principles of the Association. The theretofore hostile crowd spontaneously erupted in cheers during several parts of her address, but it was not enough to turn the tide. She was allowed to remain in the BMA, but she would have to be the last woman. That policy remained in place for two decades.

Meanwhile, Sophia Jex-Blake had, after leading a group of women to study medicine at the University of Edinburgh only to be denied the fruits of their studies at the last moment, decided to take matters into her own hands and found a medical school exclusively for women. Distinguished doctors who were incensed at the behaviour of the University of Edinburgh volunteered to teach the courses, and soon she had assembled a roster of talent that no accrediting board could deny. Garrett was initially hostile to the idea, thinking that a much more practical road was to have English women study abroad and to work for legislation to get those credentials recognised, but Jex-Blake ploughed through all difficulties, eventually sweeping Garrett into the organisation as a lecturer and administrator.

That college, the London School of Medicine for Women, would become another runaway success, educating dozens of women to enter the profession. Once medical examinations were open to women in 1877, the students of Jex-Blake's college were regular gold medal winners, sometimes scoring so much higher than their male counterparts that whole new categories of achievement needed to be created for them. Garrett served as dean and ultimately as president of the school in the late nineteenth and early twentieth centuries, raising money to meet the needs of the quickly expanding student body.

By navigating the back alleys of institutional charters, she had put herself in a position to demonstrate what women were capable of, and by founding and supporting hospitals and schools that gave women unheard of options for the care of their bodies and the education of their minds, she had worked a revolution in England's most conservative and mulish profession. When the First World War came, Britain had a trained corps of women doctors ready to serve at the front, and Elizabeth Garrett was there to wave them off. As memory and health failed her, she held on to the knowledge that all the reversals she had known had made a tangible difference. Where she had to snatch knowledge from the shadows, her professional daughters and granddaughters consumed it with relish in the full light of day, and in that realisation there was satisfaction, and peace.

FURTHER READING

Garrett's daughter, Louisa Garrett Anderson, wrote a thoroughly wonderful biography of her mother in 1939 that benefits from access to Garrett's letters and from Margaret Todd's 1918 *The Life of Sophia Jex-Blake*. Since then, Jo Manton (1987), Elizabeth Crawford (2009), and Olivia Campbell (2021) have all written engaging books about Anderson and the early fight for British women's medical education that are worth tracking down.

Chapter 10

The Path of Most Resistance

Sophia Jex-Blake and the Fight for Women's Medical Education

She had founded first England's and then Scotland's first medical school for women, and been instrumental in the passing of the Medical Act that allowed women to take the examinations for medical licensing, but by the end of her life Sophia Jex-Blake (1840–1912) was a woman living far from the centre of the movement she had honed, her opinions unheeded and her institutions either collapsed or doing their best to leave the memory of her behind.

There are few examples in the history of women in science of individuals who threw themselves so completely and readily into the public arena, forming alliances and challenging long-standing institutions with a steadfast refusal to be cowed into inaction or intimidated into silence, as that of Jex-Blake. Where others advised caution, she flew to confrontation, demanding equality and leveraging the full force of the law and public opinion to throttle the pace of progress forward. She would not wait to battle injustice, or trust in the inevitable flow of history to right systemic wrongs. Act she must, and act she did, and in the process made herself a hero to many, and a figure of primal Victorian embarrassment to not a few.

Sophia Jex-Blake had never been one for the demure road. She was a source of constant and alternating exasperation and delight to her parents, both deeply devout and social justice minded individuals who could not quite understand their high-spirited daughter. Her mother suffered from a long-standing but poorly defined illness pervaded by a nervous irritability that defined Sophia's youth. When at home, Sophia could not restrain her high-spirited ways, tumbling about, making noise, and getting into arguments for the pure intellectual fun of it. It was all too much for the nerves of her mother, and the child was sent away to boarding school time and time again, and bombarded with letters about how she could not return home until she had curbed her wickedness.

Jex-Blake's adolescence, then, was spent in the company of a revolving cast of teachers and classmates, some of whom understood and appreciated her flashes of brilliance and creativity, and others of whom took them as marks of a stubborn and unrepentant youth who must be compelled to reform. She certainly had a fast temper when contradicted, and a tendency to use her intelligence to get the better of her slower teachers in argument, which infuriated them. Fundamentally she was simply a deeply lonely child being taught to loathe her basic nature by everybody around her, who lost herself in constructing elaborate imaginary utopian societies and in attempting to bend herself to the religious orthodoxies that, surely, must change her into a good person someday – the kind her mother would take pride in and allow home again at last.

It took many years but finally, in 1857, Sophia returned home, her basic schooling completed, to consider her future and be a support to the family that was finally beginning to understand and appreciate the extent of her gifts and potential. Her mother, long her greatest critic, would, in the years that followed, grow to be her staunchest supporter, encouraging her in pursuits the mere contemplation of which would have had most Victorian mothers quailing in abject social terror. Having been a first-hand witness of so many different schools and educational systems, it was perhaps inevitable that Sophia's first inclination would be towards teaching as a profession, and that she would turn with alacrity towards the announcement that a new institution, Queen's College, had opened in London in 1858, with the goal of providing advanced instruction to the rising generation of women wishing to become professional teachers in England.

During her elementary school years, Jex-Blake had discovered in herself a love of mathematics and a particularly keen interest in mathematical puzzles. Arriving at Queen's College, she found that her mathematical skills were far in advance of her contemporaries, and she was soon offered a paid position as a tutor to a small group of students. Excited at the prospect of finally earning her own money, she wrote home to inform her parents of the offer, only to meet her father's steady refusal. As a woman from a tolerably wealthy family, he wrote, she should not consider for a moment taking pay for work such as that. She should, by all means, do the job as a means of putting her talents to good social use, but should refuse all pay for it. He could not see the importance to her of earning her own money, or the double-think he was engaging in by allowing his son to take money for working but not his daughter, and ultimately Sophia agreed in deference to his wishes to refuse payment for the current term, but to reinvestigate the issue in the future.

That disagreement notwithstanding, Sophia's life was moving forward at a promising clip when she made a fateful acquaintance. Octavia Hill was a pious, proper and brilliant woman two years Sophia's senior. To an outside observer, the two students could not have been less alike. Sophia was all sparkle, wit and motion, the brilliant daughter of a wealthy and respected family, while Octavia was the slow-moving, reclusive daughter of a single mother of greatly reduced means. Sophia was a wizard at mathematics, and Octavia had a mind for accountancy, and their relationship began in an excited mutual exchange of knowledge, and blossomed into a full and deep respect for each other's gifts and personalities.

When Sophia heard about the difficulties Octavia's family was having in finding housing, she characteristically and impulsively threw herself into the problem of solving all of her friend's difficulties for her. She suggested that she and Octavia should find a home where the two of them could live together with Octavia's family, with Sophia bearing more than her fair share of the cost. It was a generous offer that a few more moments of reflection might have suggested was doomed to failure. Octavia hated conflict and would do anything to avoid it. Sophia to some degree thrived upon it, as did Octavia's mother who was used to having her way in things. Octavia stood squarely in the middle, torn between loyalty to friend and mother, and in the end decided the only way out would be to make a clean and total break with Sophia. She would have to move out, and the friendship would have to end.

Sophia was heartbroken, struck to the core by the loss of the person she thought would be her lifetime support, her true soulmate through all of the adversities to come. She limped back home and threw herself once again into excessive religious declamations in an attempt to convince herself that, really, everything was fine, that religion, not people, was where true happiness was to be had, and that love of Jesus would cure all her ills. She was not fooling anyone, however, and the depth of the hurt demanded a new thrust of action to keep her from lingering over her wounds. She resolved that the next step in her education would be to seek a position at a school in Germany, France, or the United States, to learn how other countries educated their children. Her father vetoed France out of fear that she would turn Catholic, and her mother the United States because of the distance involved, and so she went to Germany, where she arrived and presented herself at a school which had already told her it had no position for her, confident that her pluck and determination would win her a job somehow.

It did. She experienced all of the ups and downs of a new teacher – the self doubt that comes with feeling you do not know the topic well enough to teach it, the agony over having to discipline students, and the frustration of dealing with children who took pains to make fun of her every mistake, clothing choice and cultural difference. These were tough times, but she had learned from her fellow teachers the value of mutual religious tolerance, which went far to taking the edge off her self-righteous upbringing, and stored away details of school organisation that would come in handy in her great educational pursuits of mid-life.

As of yet, medicine as a career had not remotely entered Sophia Jex-Blake's mind. She wanted to devote herself to designing and running a new school with her family's resources, and in 1865 travelled to the United States to survey educational theories and institutions there. It was on this trip that she met Lucy Sewall, the resident physician at the New England Hospital for Women and Children, which had been founded in 1862 by Marie Zakrzewska after her time with the Blackwell sisters. Sophia was thus thrust into the centre of the women's medical movement in the United States, and met its leading figures as they heroically built up the institutions to support women's medical training and practice from the bare ground.

These were heady surroundings, and Sophia found that, at the end of her tour of American colleges, the desire to return to England as a teacher had been overwritten by a need to participate in the cause of women's medicine. She worked at the New England Hospital as an accountant and aide, while picking up the rudiments of the trade, and intended to attend Blackwell's new school in New York to begin her formal training, when the death of her father recalled her to England.

After recovering from her father's passing, Jex-Blake began formulating plans for her British medical education. The only other British woman who had successfully obtained a licence as a practising medical doctor was Elizabeth Garrett Anderson, who as we learned last chapter had used a loophole in 1865 to take a valid medical examination from the Society of Apothecaries. Her route to a qualifying exam was closed instantly after she obtained it, and since then the medical community had closed ranks to prevent future female aspirants from following her example.

Jex-Blake, therefore, had to find a new path to medical education. During some time spent in Edinburgh gathering information about educational practices, she had been favourably impressed by their relative progressivism, and so decided to begin her campaign at the University of Edinburgh in 1869, beginning thereby four of the hardest but most rewarding years of her life. Her opponent during these years was Sir Robert Christison, an eminent physician who was vehemently opposed to the idea of women receiving a medical education. At every step of her harrowing experience fighting for the right to learn, Christison would be there, mobilising his official power and unofficial influence to foil her. After the ultimate failure of her first application, she gathered a core group of six other women interested in a medical education. Collectively known as the Edinburgh Seven, they were to suffer indignities and setbacks of shameful scale in the coming years.

Their application to the university once approved, they had to find a way to learn under the staggering series of restrictions that had been placed on their acceptance. There were some classes from which they were simply banned, but even in those allowed to them, they had to appeal to the professors to form a separate class just for them because the male students protested vigorously at the idea of being forced to sit in the same classroom as women students. Since those separate classes were so much smaller in size, they were correspondingly more expensive, and more often than not it was Sophia Jex-Blake who had to make up the difference from her own pocket. Upon their first examinations, several of the Seven earned top scores that would ordinarily have entitled them to prizes for academic distinction – which were of course refused them – which bred so much resentment among the male students who saw themselves beaten so soundly that they lent an increasingly ready ear to professors like Christison who urged that the ladies' lives be made as unpleasant as possible.

The Seven began having to walk to classes together to avoid being accosted by male students, and even then had to bear verbal insults to and from class and regular pelting with garbage from students who felt that education was their right and theirs alone, all culminating in the Surgeons' Hall Riot of 1870. The women were due to take an anatomy exam when they found a large crowd barring their way, with Dr Christison's assistant leading the mob as they threatened the ladies trying to enter Surgeons' Hall. Stones and refuse were thrown at them and they were only rescued from further physical violence by a group of students who forced the doors open for them and conducted them to the examination hall, where they took their exam in spite of another group of students having thrust a sheep into the room to further disrupt them.

The Surgeons' Hall Riot was the high-water mark of the physical intimidation of the Edinburgh Seven, but as much as they had gained sympathy as a result of it, their administrative woes were far from over. No sooner would they win one right than complicated wrangling in the upper echelons of the university would wrest it away from them again. Christison and his phalanx of traditionalists expertly appealed each victory until they obtained the results they wanted, and by 1873 the university declared that, even if the women managed to take all the necessary classes (which they largely had thanks to Edinburgh's extra-mural system) and obtain the necessary ward experience (which had been made as difficult as possible by the Royal Infirmary's restrictions on their attendance at the hospital), they still would not be allowed to take a medical degree.

The Edinburgh campaign was over. Jex-Blake had staked her reputation on combating the academic system through every legal and public means at her disposal, tirelessly collecting allies, signatures and legal opinions at the expense of her own studies, and in the end it had not been enough. The Seven broke up to further their education elsewhere, while Jex-Blake, more convinced than ever of the rightness of her cause, planned to move the fight to London itself and the halls of parliament.

Transplanted to London, Jex-Blake combined her gift for organisation with her years of educational observation to set about the dual task of establishing a new medical school for women and to provide information to lawmakers about the progress and obstacles faced by women doctors around the world. She and Elizabeth Garrett Anderson disagreed fundamentally on how the cause of women doctors was best served – Jex-Blake favoured aggressive legislative lobbying and appeal to the courts while Anderson thought women should get their degrees in Europe and practise unlicensed in Britain until the establishment deigned to take notice of the good work they did – but both put aside their differences long enough to found the London School of Medicine for Women in 1875. Jex-Blake did most of the organising and planning for the school while Anderson reluctantly lent her name to the cause to avoid the appearance of dissent in the medical ranks. Likewise in politics it was Jex-Blake who paid visits to politicians, providing them with facts and figures from her correspondents in the United States and her time in Edinburgh to prove women's capacity for medical work. As a result, members of parliament proposed a series of bills which, after several bitter defeats, resulted in 1876 in an Act which enabled all universities to award degrees to women if they so chose.

Ireland took the lead in taking advantage of the new bill, and it was there that the first British women, Jex-Blake included, took their qualifying exams to become, at long last, licensed doctors. This should have been the beginning of a new dawn for Jex-Blake's career, with the London School booming and her degree finally in hand, but instead it was the moment that saw Jex-Blake progressively and insistently shunted to the sidelines of the movement she had risked so much to see succeed. She was passed over for the position of Acting Secretary of the London School because her personality, which had been perfectly suited to a new school struggling to find its way, was deemed too volatile for an established and thriving institution.

She returned to Edinburgh and there founded the Edinburgh School of Medicine while concurrently developing her own practice and a dispensary for the poor. Once again, initial success gave way to frustration as Jex-Blake demonstrated an inflexibility as a school administrator, which drove several students into establishing a rival school whose connections to a more prestigious intern hospital (in fact the same one that Jex-Blake had spent voluminous energy trying to open to women in the early 1870s) attracted students away from the Edinburgh School. In 1898, the school closed, and the following year Jex-Blake moved to a small farm in Sussex with one of her students, Margaret Todd, to enjoy a serene retirement far from the struggles that she had given over so much of her life to undertaking.

There she happily oversaw the workers bringing in the yearly harvest, enjoyed visits from a steadily decreasing number of old friends, and took a daily carriage ride that she often fell asleep in the middle of, all while the women's medical profession forged steadily on, remembering her only now and then but resolutely taking no heed of her occasional and dwindling advice. Sophia Jex-Blake died on 7 January 1912, among her last words a piece of characteristically thoughtful advice to her companion Ms. Todd, who was watching over her, 'Now do go and have a good rest.'

The Edinburgh Seven were awarded posthumous degrees by the University of Edinburgh in July 2019.

Further Reading

The main source for the life and work of Jex-Blake is Margaret Todd's classic biography of her, *The Life of Sophia Jex-Blake* (1918), which you can find in inexpensive reprint editions, but I probably would not recommend that unless you are a serious Jex-Blake enthusiast. The wealth of letters and diary entries it provides are great sources for those who want a deep dive into her personality, but are probably on the dense side for those who are taking their first pass through her life. For those, I would say *Sophia Jex-Blake: A Woman Pioneer in Nineteenth-Century Medical Reform* (1993) by Shirley Roberts is your best bet. Extensively based on Todd's book, it is a much smoother account which is more selective in the original sources it quotes.

Chapter 11

The Experimentalist

The Tale of Mary Putnam Jacobi vs. Proper Victorian Medicine

As we have seen, the nineteenth century boasts a rich roster of medical women, any one of whom is the stuff of heroes: the trailblazing Blackwell sisters; the cautious Elizabeth Garrett Anderson; the firebrand Sophia Jex-Blake; the rigorous Marie Zakrzewska; the peace-keeping Lucy Sewall. Any one of them deserves all the attention our fractured post-modern consciousnesses can spare, but personally, my utmost favourite has always been the most complicated figure in that gifted pantheon – Dr Mary Putnam Jacobi (1842–1906).

Jacobi was a figure of astonishing intellect and aggressive bravery who brooked no nonsense in the pursuit of medical truth. She was a revolutionary even among revolutionaries, spurned equally by large swathes of the male medical establishment for being a woman and by the nascent women's medical movement for being too devoted to laboratory work and original research. Only by her life's end was she accepted for what she was: a pioneer in applying microscopic and chemical analysis to the treatment of patients, but the road to that acceptance was anything but a steady one.

Mary Putnam, the oldest of eleven children, could have chosen any path for her life. She was born the daughter of G. P. Putnam, one of the most influential publishers in nineteenth-century America, whose home was regularly visited by some of the era's most famous writers, including Frederika Bremer and Susan Warner. Inspired by her interactions with such renowned, independent and intellectually stimulating women, Putnam determined to make her living as a writer, and started writing brief moral essays and stories at the age of 9.

Under the progressive influence of her family and circle of acquaintances, Putnam began calling standard gender roles into question. Attending Twelfth Street School in New York, she wrote an essay that took a prompt about William the Conqueror and changed it into a piece about the need to move away from meekness and passivity as the feminine ideal. If women were to become all they might be, she stated, they had to start valuing new virtues, like self-sufficiency and a thorough sense of responsibility that refused to surrender control of one's life in exchange for mere comfort.

With her senses attuned to historical structures that enforce a cult of feminine passivity and obedience, it was inevitable that young Putnam would come into conflict with the Baptist faith of her family. She recorded her doubts, both about the inconsistencies of dogma and the historically poor record of established religion with regard to women and reason, and met with a Baptist cleric regularly in the hopes that he could show her a way back to faith. He could not, however, and his total inability to come up with reasonable answers to basic questions, coupled with his insistence on criticising her as 'unwomanly' for questioning the roles the church had decreed for her, resolved her to renounce her membership of the First Baptist Church in 1863. She decided that, if there were truths to existence to be discovered, they would come not from the wisdom of Bronze Age patriarchal elders, but from an open and active investigation into natural phenomena.

For some years before her renunciation of Baptist religion, Putnam had been gaining, here and there as the opportunities presented themselves, instruction in medicine. She attended lectures and dissections, and spent time with the women's medicine pioneer Elizabeth Blackwell, who in 1847 had been the first woman to attend medical school in the United States and had, in 1857, founded the New York Infirmary for Women and Children with her sister Emily. By Putnam's time, most universities had closed off any loopholes like those that allowed Blackwell to attend, and so Putnam was compelled to study instead at the New York College of Pharmacy.

Studying at a pharmacy college instead of a more traditional medical school was the route being charted by Elizabeth Garrett Anderson simultaneously in England, and it was to have a profound influence on how Putnam approached medicine. She studied the preparation of medications and their chemistry, which gave her a more molecular view of disease and its remedy than was available to more traditional medical students. In March 1863, she graduated from the New York College of Pharmacy and, after a brief stint as a medical volunteer on the front lines during the Civil War, she attended one of the only two schools offering medical training to women: the Female Medical College of Pennsylvania.

Her time in Pennsylvania was to prove a source of frustration for all concerned. Putnam was frustrated at the slow pace of the courses and the low quality of her fellow students. She applied to graduate early without having taken all the courses required for graduation, stating that her previous work at the College of Pharmacy and the strength of her thesis paper should be enough qualification, and that she could not possibly learn anything of value from the rambling and elementary courses the school was trying to compel her to take. Administrators were riled by the impertinence of her request and its suggestion that their standards of instruction were so low as to be beneath consideration for a student of actual talent. Nevertheless, they ultimately approved her graduation in 1864, and Putnam had her second medical degree in as many years.

Her time at Philadelphia, however, had definitively shown her that the United States was not the place to study for a woman who actually wanted to learn the details of medical practice, and especially the craft of experimental medical research. So, in 1866, she turned to Paris to truly complete her education. Influenced heavily by the cellular approach to medical research pioneered by Rudolf Virchow in the 1850s, the Parisian medical scene was the perfect place to be for a molecularly-orientated young doctor like Putnam, and she threw herself not only into her studies, but into the heady political climate of late 1860s France.

These were the last years of Napoleon III's mixed attempt to realise for France a new empire, when democratic and socialist ideas ran rampant among the educated classes who bridled under Napoleon's steady curtailing of expressive freedoms. Putnam fell in naturally with progressive-thinking families and intellectuals, remaining in Paris during the lean times following the fall of Napoleon in the Franco-Prussian War and experiencing the bracing but doomed culturo-political moment that was the Paris Commune.

Her main work for the half decade of her Paris residency, however, was the slow and sure execution of her plan to gain entrance to the prestigious École de Medicine. She worked in the laboratory of Antoine Ranvier, himself the assistant to Claude Bernard, originator of the concept of biological homeostasis. She wrote essays for American publications describing French scientific and political life. She worked at the Salpêtrière clinic gaining insight into neurological theory. By 1868, she had such a wide array of degrees, experiences and contacts that the École de Medicine felt it could not legitimately prevent her from attending classes, and on 25 January she walked into the medical amphitheatre there for the first time, though the achievement was muted somewhat by having to enter through a side door and sit in a specially appointed chair.

Putnam graduated in July 1871 in a Paris that was slowly piecing itself together after the dramatic collapse of the Commune, and moved back to New York shortly thereafter to begin charting an entirely new course for women medical doctors. By 1871, several women doctors were well known to the public and established in various practices and institutions, but by and large their approach to medical practice was centred more around patient care than experimental research. The predominantly male medical establishment was hard-pressed enough to find it in themselves to admit women doctors when those doctors approached their work in a reassuringly motherly manner, but a woman regularly performing tissue dissections, chemical analysis and vivisections was a creature of such unwomanly interests as to be beyond comprehension, a being of horror even to other women doctors.

Putnam set up a small office in New York upon her return and began publishing accounts of her medical findings in the *Medical Record.* She believed strongly in the value of what was then called nutrition as a means of evaluating and fostering health. For the late nineteenth century, 'nutrition' was about the investigation of how cells take in and break down chemicals in their cycle of birth, renewal and death. Approaching disease from the perspective of the chemicals needed to nourish and sustain cells, Putnam (who became Mary Putnam Jacobi upon marrying the esteemed Dr Abraham Jacobi in 1873) was able to view the workings of illnesses from a foundation-up perspective which allowed her to devise new experiments and medical procedures.

This cellular perspective put her in a position to appreciate the emerging theory of bacteriology while more traditional doctors like her husband or Elizabeth Blackwell fought against the idea that diseases could be caused by germs. Doctors attached to social reform movements particularly viewed bacteriology with mistrust. They believed diseases were caused by social and behavioural problems, and resisted any notion that a pathogen which struck rich and poor, virtuous and depraved alike, could be the root cause. Putnam made it part of her life's work to publicise the findings of the rising bacteriology researchers, particularly after the death of her oldest child at the hands of diphtheria.

Putnam wrote 120 scientific papers over the course of her career, but none brought her the same degree of fame as 1876's *The Question of Rest for Women During Menstruation*, written in the wake of the publication in 1875 of Edward Clarke's now infamous *Sex in Education; or a Fair Chance for the Girls*. Clarke, a retired Harvard professor, claimed that intellectual work un-womanised women and rendered them infertile. He believed that the reproductive and nervous systems were fundamentally linked, and that resources diverted towards one could only come at the cost of the other. You want to read a difficult book? That's fine, but it will take 2 units of resources away from your uterus. You want to be active during menstruation? All right, but it will leave you in chronic pain.

Putnam found Clarke's work reactive and fundamentally unscientific, and proceeded gathering data about what actually happens to women, both on a psychological and cellular level, during the process of menstruation. She used her 1876 paper and subsequent 1877 book to demonstrate that, on the basis of the statistical data she gathered and chemical analyses she had performed, the women who experience the least pain during menstruation are not those who have removed themselves from all physical and intellectual effort, but precisely those who had a robust childhood and who continue to challenge themselves mentally and physically. On the basis of this data, she argued strenuously for more girls' physical education programmes, and the expansion of educational and occupational opportunities for women as a means of saving their health from the dangers of a socially and religiously mandated torpor.

Her life was one of struggle, for women against the inherited advice of medical Victorianism, for bacteriology in the face of established social behaviour medicine, for women's suffrage during its darkest era, and, most controversially, as virtually the only woman to argue publicly for the continued use of vivisection in medical research amidst the great anti-vivisectionist movement of the late nineteenth and early twentieth centuries. This last crusade is in many ways her most intriguing, the one it is hardest to come to a firm and fast opinion about (at least for me). On the one hand, from the point of view of a theoretically more advanced twenty-first-century sense of empathy, it is easy to see the anti-vivisectionists as the heroes, striking a blow for a more humane treatment of other species at the hands of an often luxuriously wasteful medical community that dealt out untellable amounts of suffering for often undetectable amounts of benefit.

But on the other hand, there is the figure of Putnam herself, a hard-as-nails scientist who believed that, to do things right and actually understand what is happening on a functional level, one must do certain experiments, and who was willing to do the bloody business of performing them herself amidst almost universal disgust that a woman should be so grotesque as to willingly perform such labours. She could have moved into other parts of medicine, she could have carried out her experiments but stayed away from the public stage, but she cared so little for reputation when set in the balance against advocating for what she deemed necessary for the advancement of medicine and science that she chose the long, bloody, hard path to notoriety, and there is something in that determination that is compelling even if its object is morally tendentious.

Her comments before Congress in 1900 against a proposed anti-vivisection bill were among Putnam's last public acts. In 1896, she developed the first symptoms of a brain tumour that would ultimately take her life a decade later, and after pushing on with her work as best she could for some years, she decided to limit her responsibilities and throw herself into a complete documentation of her own case, including her heart-rending accounts of the slow loss of the two things she had always been able to count on in life: her mental sharpness and her force of will. She died on 10 June 1906, having done all that could be asked of her in one life to secure access to an intellectually and physically stimulating life for women, a future in experimental medicine for women doctors, and a cellularly-centred path forward for medicine generally. Fierce in opposition, fearless in alliance, too complicated to be a popular hero, but too deserving to be forgotten, everything about her was intensity and struggle, and it is seemingly unlikely we shall soon see her type again.

Further Reading

Mary Putnam Jacobi & The Politics of Medicine in Nineteenth-Century America (2009) by Carla Bittel is the book to get. It bears some of the marks of its time, including a tendency to use the word 'perform' in variously eccentric ways that was the particular fad of the first decade of twenty-first-century academia, but it thoroughly investigates all the many aspects of Putnam's many-faceted career, including her role in bringing high society into the suffragette fold in the late nineteenth century.

Chapter 12

One Woman Against The Black Death

The Saga of Dr Edith Pechey-Phipson and The Fight for Medical Women in India

In 1896, the city of Bombay recorded its first case of bubonic plague, a disease which would grow to claim 10 million lives over the following decade as the government stumbled after a consistent health policy to combat the bacterium. At the outset of the epidemic, as doctors were warning the government that the dreaded Black Death of medieval infamy was eating into the heart of Britain's Imperial showcase city, the government, in a move depressingly familiar to people possessing an intact memory of 2020, decided to waste crucial months downplaying the existence of the disease at the request of Bombay's merchants so as not to upset the city's trade.

While the Advocate of India declared flatly that there was no bubonic plague in India, a doctor who had gained renown as the motivating force behind women's medical education in India took up her pen and, in the pages of the *Bombay Gazette*, lambasted the government for its economically motivated inaction, and its continued inability to coordinate a sensible response for the disease clearly in their midst, claiming nearly 2,000 lives a week in Bombay alone. She was Dr Edith Pechey-Phipson (1845–1908), and at the time of the Bombay Plague she was entering her third decade of compelling medical authorities – through the power of her words and example – to re-evaluate the underpinnings of their theories and policies.

Pechey had burst into the British consciousness in 1869 as a member of the group organised by Sophia Jex-Blake variously known as the Edinburgh Five or the Edinburgh Seven depending on who you decide to count as 'in' the group. This was the group of young women organised by Jex-Blake who sought to study medicine at the University of Edinburgh, and who would spend the next four years fighting every manner of institutional obstructionism in an ultimately futile attempt to gain the degrees that their work had entitled them to. Physically threatened by male students who were being actively encouraged by reactionary professors, emotionally battered and academically stonewalled, the women emerged from their four-year ordeal with a solid but dearly bought foundation of medical knowledge and a deep scepticism about the ability of institutions to reform themselves in addressing long-standing structural problems.

Pechey was perhaps the group's most persuasive writer and orator, her letters to the newspapers instrumental in evoking sympathy for the uneven battle being waged by the seven medical hopefuls, and her speeches a mixture of unanswerable logic and undeniable emotional impact. While Jex-Blake's multiple duties in confronting the university administration while attempting to continue her own education stretched her to a state of mental and emotional fatigue that had an understandable way of creeping into her public statements, Pechey had the gift of somehow being able to tell people exactly what they did not want to hear, and compelling them to take action to correct it – a skill that would serve her well in getting India's first all-woman-staffed hospital up and running a decade later.

Pechey was also the star student in the group, claiming a first place in chemistry that would have won her a Hope scholarship were it not for her professor's concern that the male students would not respond well to having it pointed out that they had, to a man, been bested intellectually by a woman. That scholarship was awarded to a male student who had performed less well than Pechey, but the renewed example of the university's lack of fair play with regard to its women students evoked yet more public sympathy and discussion.

The Seven did not, however, gain their medical degrees at Edinburgh, but rather broke up in 1873 when their forward progress was definitively barred by a combination of university bodies, each controlled at least in part by the influence of Sir Robert Christison, who was determined to use every shred of prestige and power at his disposal to suppress entirely women's access to medical education. Jex-Blake, having lost the battle, decided to enlarge the scale of the conflict, and took the case of women's education to London, where she simultaneously worked for the establishment of a women's medical college (which opened as the London School of Medicine for Women in 1874 and for which Pechey gave the inaugural address) and for acts of parliament that would compel universities to allow women to take the examinations that would grant them medical degrees.

Theoretically, until women could obtain such degrees, they could not openly practise as doctors in England. The only two women doctors currently practising legally in the country, Elizabeth Blackwell and Elizabeth Garrett Anderson, had gained their licences to work as doctors before the loopholes barring women's medical practice had been closed off, and since 1862 they possessed no successor.

No LEGAL successor, that is, for lacking the ability to obtain a legal licence to practise because of governmental and institutional prejudice, many women decided to simply carry on with their medical work, licence be damned. Among those women was Edith Pechey. In 1875, Pechey took up the position of house surgeon at the Birmingham and Midlands Hospital for Women, a job previously held by Dr Louisa Atkins, who had also been operating without a medical licence since her MD, received at the University of Zurich in 1872, was not recognised by British medical licensing laws. Pechey held the post for a year, working at the time with Dr Lawson B. Tait, who was an early advocate of using disinfectants in surgical procedures, including the radical notion that surgeons should vigorously wash their hands with soap and water between operations. A hallmark of Pechey's work as a doctor from that time forward was a thorough belief in the germ theory of disease, the utility of disinfectants, and the need to keep constantly aware of the newest theories of safe surgical practice, all of which came into play when she began designing her own hospital procedures in India.

In the winter of 1876, after several failed campaigns to compel British authorities and universities to move forward on giving women a viable and official path to obtain medical degrees, Pechey and Jex-Blake, along with Annie Clark, travelled to the University of Bern to study for the medical examinations there. On 31 January 1877, Pechey took and passed her medical examination and earned the MD that proved the depth of her knowledge, but meant precisely nothing to the British licensing authorities who had the previous decade closed off foreign diplomas as a route women could take to creating a medical practice in England.

After receiving her MD, Pechey elected to take the road advocated by Elizabeth Garrett Anderson – to practise in England without a licence and, by conspicuously demonstrating her competence, to become another living data point compelling change in British medicine. From 1877 to 1883 she practised privately in Leeds while lecturing on medical topics throughout England and taking part in the Medical Women's Federation of England, of which she was elected president in 1882.

Private practice and public educational advocacy – such might have been the overall trajectory of her life had E. G. Anderson not mentioned her to George Kittredge, a philanthropist and reformer who had created the Medical Women for India Fund and was currently seeking a woman doctor to head a new hospital in Bombay to be staffed entirely by women. This hospital, the brainchild of Kittredge and Sorabjee Shapoorjee Bengallee, was to be funded by a generous grant from Pestonji Hormusji Cama and would come to be known as the Cama Hospital. It was created to respond to a desperate need in Indian society, recognised by the visionary Indian reformer Behramji Malabari (1854–1912), to improve women's education in India and to recognise and provide for their medical needs.

Pechey agreed to Kittredge's proposal to become head physician at the proposed Cama Hospital, and arrived in Bombay in 1883 where she would spend the next years experiencing the full brunt of Indian bureaucratic inertia, that particular amalgam of British and local practice that ensured that every request, no matter how miniscule, wandered with unspeakable lethargy up every rung of government, pushed on its way by officials who dreaded more than anything having to be responsible for being on record as having made a decision about something. *Everything* about the hospital and its associated dispensary had to wend its way through this ponderous labyrinth, but through an almost unfathomable patience she was able to put in place a staff, a nurse's training programme, admission procedures, a system for obtaining medicine and furnishings, and facilities that catered to the various cultural demands of India's population.

Demand for the services of the hospital and dispensary constantly overpowered the ability of Pechey and her small staff to supply it, as women from all levels of society, many of whom had been denied any thoroughgoing medical attention on account of strict rules forbidding certain women from being examined in any but the most indirect fashion by male doctors, flocked to a hospital known to be staffed entirely by women boasting the most modern medical educations. Some time previously, Bombay University and Grant Medical College had opened their doors to women students, and as they began to graduate, they assumed leadership roles not only in Cama, but in new organisations springing up throughout India, inspired by the success of Cama to meet a clear cultural and medical need.

Pechey held her position at Cama until 1894 when she at last retired, physically worn out by a job that consumed virtually every hour of every day and the deleterious effects of encroaching diabetes compounded by the constant strain of living and working in India's extreme heat. During that time, she took every opportunity to promote the expansion of Indian girls' and women's education, and to speak out against practices that limited Indian women's ability to determine the course of their own life, particularly the joint policies of child marriage and enforced widowhood that could see a girl married at age 12 to a man in his sixties, who upon dying perhaps two years later thereby condemned his now 14-year-old bride to live the rest of her life as a perpetual widow of socially low regard whose sustenance was dependent on the vagaries of her relatives' good will.

She vigorously undertook the defence of Rukhmabai, a child bride who refused to obey the summons of her husband to live with him when she turned 17 and took her case to court, thereby creating a national scandal that polarised the traditional and progressive elements of Indian society. After Rukhmabai won that case, Pechey collected funds to allow her to travel to England to study at the London School of Medicine, and when she returned, Pechey arranged to have her serve as house surgeon at Cama Hospital for six months on her way to becoming chief medical officer at Surat's women's hospital for the following two decades.

Though she had retired on grounds of exhaustion in 1894, Pechey dipped into her substantial reserves of energy to meet the Bombay Plague crisis in 1896, not only using her fame and knowledge to educate the public about the real state of the disease and the government's failures in responding to it but serving on the staff of the Cutchi-Memon Plague Hospital, as well as on house-to-house medical inspection teams, while pressing insistently against cultural prejudices for the adoption of a vaccine developed by cholera hero Dr Waldemar Haffkine that proved remarkably effective in combating the disease.

Having done her duty to use her medical knowledge to combat an epidemic with every means at her disposal and every reserve of her strength, she retired at last and definitively with the diminution of the plague's ferocity, and returned to England with her husband (a merchant who had been a driving force in the sustaining of Cama hospital whom she had married in 1889). There she contributed her voice to the next great fight, that for women's suffrage, where in spite of suffering from breast cancer and diabetes she managed, as one of her last public acts, to participate at the head of the famous 1907 London Mud March, a display of 3,000 women in support of a new suffrage bill, which in turn inspired the following year's Women's Sunday. That gathering of half a *million* suffrage supporters took place in June 1908, two months after the death of Dr Edith Pechey-Phipson, the woman who four decades before had dared to ask for an education, and who had since educated the world by her example.

Further Reading

Edythe Lutzker's 1973 *Edith Pechey-Phipson MD: The Story of England's Foremost Pioneering Woman Doctor* will probably be your best source for Edith Pechey for a while. It gives absolutely minute detail about the tremendous bureaucratic and institutional muck that Pechey had to wade through both as a member of the Edinburgh Seven and as head of Cama Hospital. Accounts of resolutions and counter-directives and chains of bureaucratic decrees is, granted, not the most exciting reading, but it is tremendously important to comprehending the forces aligned against Pechey, and makes her eventual success all the more impressive. The book also strikes a good balance (particularly for the time) of paying heed to medical best practices while recognising that Western moral judgments can and did get conflated with medical judgments and policy in a manner not always easy to tease apart.

Chapter 13

The Totally Improbable, Completely True Life of Betsi Cadwaladr, Welsh War Nurse

On a winter's night in 1854, two steel-willed women regarded each other with mutual dislike across a desk located on a scrap of misery-soaked land. Two more different people there could not have been: the younger, in her mid-thirties, was the daughter of a privileged house who had studied nursing against her family's wishes, and was now attempting to instil some order in the midst of the chaos of war. Her name was Florence Nightingale, the Crimean War's 'Lady with the Lamp'. The older, in her mid-sixties, was a Welshwoman who had travelled the world as a servant to various ship captains, experiencing adventure, peril and destitution in just about equal quantities. She often gave her name as Elizabeth Davis, but she was born Betsi Cadwaladr (1789–1860), and she had never in her life backed down from a fight.

In their confrontation, all the power and authority, the resources and social standing, lay with Nightingale, but Cadwaladr was possessed of a singular soul that would not cower before power when she felt a wrong was being done. She thought Nightingale's use of her nurses, and her distribution of provisions, were woefully misguided and causing unnecessary suffering for the Crimean War's manifold victims, and said so. She fumed that she, as a nurse with a decade's worth of experience, was being kept on shirt-mending duty when her skills were desperately needed in the General Hospital at Balaclava tending to wounded men.

Nightingale, worn to the nub already with the gigantic task of creating something like a hospital from the pit of suffering that was Scutari, and now having to deal with this opinionated Welshwoman on top of everything else, washed her hands of the whole business. 'I have done with you *entirely*,' Nightingale said in exasperation as she gave the old woman leave to do what she would, and with that Cadwaladr headed for Balaclava and the hardest years of her life.

Betsi Cadwaladr and Hardship had walked long in each other's company by that point. She was never sure what year she was born, but knew that her mother died when she was but 5 years old, leaving her to the care of her preacher father and her cruel older sister. An impetuous child who loved dancing, she was fiercely beaten whenever she was caught doing it. She ran away from home at the age of 9, and then ran away from her second home at the age of 14, making her way to the big city of Liverpool with no particular plan for how to support herself once there.

She was, however, gifted with the astounding ability of making friends wherever she went, and the improbable luck of finding kinsfolk in every corner of the world willing to help her on to her next stage in life. Arriving in Liverpool, she applied to become a domestic servant and proved her worth early when, given sole charge of a shop one day, she noticed somebody breaking a pane of glass and reaching in through the window to try and steal a bolt of cloth. This country child just arrived in the city did not run screaming, or duck into the nearest closet to hide. No, she did what she would always do in life when faced with injustice, springing instinctively to action. She grabbed a nearby pole and beat the thief's hand away then flung open the door, chased the man down on foot, tackled him, and pummelled him into submission until the police arrived to take him into custody.

A message had thus been sent to the cosmos: *Do Not Mess With Betsi Cadwaladr.*

Soon even the bustling city life of Liverpool became too small for Cadwaladr and she signed on as a servant on a series of trading ships bound for exotic ports. She visited China and stumbled by accident into the emperor's council chambers, and was nearly executed on the spot as a result. She rode elephants and dined in palaces while escorting high-caste Burmese ladies. She was kidnapped by a former prince desperate to marry her, and nearly stabbed to death by another whose pomposities she had dared to laugh at. She walked across a bridge made up of an entire fleet of merchant ships while carrying a delighted Brazilian princess in her arms. Her quick thinking saved two ships from going down to the bottom of the ocean, and her striking looks, unbreakable honesty and fierce spirit had prompted a dozen men to propose to her in vain.

Returning to England at last, she had amassed a small fortune from her own efforts at trading, and in gifts from grateful royalty and passengers whom she had found ways to aid along their way. Receiving her back pay, she left her valuable possessions on her boat, and proceeded to look for ways to invest her new-found capital. And that is when, for the first but not last time, she lost everything. She put all of her earnings into the purchase of some rental properties which, it turned out, the seller did not actually own. Her money lost in a scam, she at least had her stored-up valuables. Returning to the port, she found, however, that the ship had left without bothering to put her goods back on shore.

Cadwaladr had served well and faithfully for years, had rejected marriage offers from princes and captains, and was now right back where she started, broke in England, without any prospect of financial security in her approaching old age. But she was made of stern stuff, and simply set her shoulder to the wheel again, finding employment as a servant in a series of homes culminating in work with a great and prosperous lawyer named in her memoir only as 'Mr H'. She served as both nurse and servant, and his gratitude for all she did for him was so great that he willed the majority of his substantial estate to her, the document being signed by his hand and witnessed by two people of good standing.

When he eventually passed, Cadwaladr's future should again have been secured, but the lawyer's relations descended en masse and declared the will void for having only two witnesses instead of three. Already provided for in Mr H's will, the family decided to take Cadwaladr's share of his estate as well, leaving her once again without employment or financial reserves for the future. No longer young, she had to face the prospect of starting life from scratch, yet again.

Which is precisely when the grandly disastrous cavalcade of international posturing known as the Crimean War broke out, in 1853. In the gnash of Russia trying to assert itself in the Balkans, Napoleon III trying to claim a small slice of the military legacy that was his uncle's, and England getting its oar in, around 750,000 men were killed or wounded. British battlefield medicine, still resolutely stuck in the age of the Duke of Wellington, was woefully unprepared for the scale of suffering hurled its way from the Crimean battlefields. Reports of understaffed hospitals, reeking with the dread stench of infection, stuffed with the dead and dying, reached England and prompted a furore that led Florence Nightingale and a squadron of supporting nurses to offer their services.

Betsi Cadwaladr took note of the nursing drive and, having herself been nurse to a variety of ailing patrons, knew she could be of value. Too late to join Nightingale's first detachment of nurses, she secured a position with the next group out under Mary Stanley. Arriving at Scutari, Nightingale's main base of operations, she was frustrated from the first. Instead of using her years of experience in both nursing and resource management (she had been in regular charge of ship loading and inventory during her years on merchant vessels), she was employed as a seamstress, explicitly forbidden from even talking to the wounded. She also bristled under Nightingale's policy for distributing the Free Gifts sent from England for the soldiers. Cadwaladr saw storehouses full of linen and food, rotting away instead of being put to the soldiers' use, because Nightingale's requisition system was too formal and unbending to allow nurses to use their insight to distribute these resources as needed.

Nightingale was of course labouring under the immense task of setting a critically broken system aright, juggling the tasks of head nurse, resource administrator, fund distributor, public building designer, and parliamentary correspondent – all in circumstances of omnipresent suffering and death. To be fair, Cadwaladr probably could have done better in seeing all the things Nightingale was doing right instead of honing in on the few things she had yet to figure out, but as always in her life, the presence of injustice got her blood up, and when it came time to talk to Nightingale directly, she had nothing good to say about The Lady with the Lamp or her methods of administration.

Transferred closer to the front at Balaclava General Hospital, Cadwaladr set about reforming the hospital as she thought best, hounding the requisitions officers until she got the food, bedding, forks, knives, bandages, toothbrushes and clothing that her charges desperately needed. Army provisioners who could count on Nightingale to follow the rules for distribution were bowled back on their heels by the force of nature that was Betsi Cadwaladr. She worked in the special kitchen during the day, preparing meals, while intermittently touring the wards she had reorganised, personally removing literally bucketfuls of maggots from the flesh of patients who had been left too long unattended by the couple of doctors working the hospital. Under her care, patients' wounds were cleaned and bandaged, their food needs carefully monitored, and the necessary provisions for a semi-comfortable stay acquired.

Doing a similar multitude of jobs back at Scutari, the young Florence Nightingale worked herself into an invalid state that would remain with her for the next fifty years of life. Cadwaladr was thirty years older, doing the same work, and doing it closer to the war front, and in spite of a lifetime accustomed to hard labour, she too faced inevitable breakdown. Cholera and dysentery both dug their claws deep into her sexagenarian frame, and in 1855 she was forced to return to England.

Her original contract had stipulated that nurse wages were set at a starting amount of 10 shillings a week, with raises up to 25*s* depending on the quality of service done. Nightingale, when accepting Cadwaladr's resignation, only offered her the 10-shilling rate when settling up her back wages in spite of her Herculean efforts at Balaclava. Cadwaladr, however, knew her worth, and was not about to take the rate reserved for drunken and incompetent nurses as the wages for her health-breaking heroics. Nightingale compromised, and they settled at 18 shillings a week.

Returning to England, Cadwaladr was 66 years old, in ill health, without a job, and carrying a few thin pounds of money by way of reward for her service to the British army. She wrote her memoirs with the help of a historian by the name of Jane Williams, which were published in 1857 and which end on an appeal crushing in its desperation:

> Notice
> In the decline of life, the Heroine of this narrative is left unprovided for.
>
> She is anxious to obtain employment in some public institution, and is fully capable of executing any office of trust and vigilant inspection.
>
> Benevolent readers who may wish to contribute to the comfort of her latter years, can pay in subscriptions for her, either to Mr Murgatroyd, 18, Stafford Row, Pimlico, or to Mr John Brown, 9, Hans Place, Sloane Street.

After a life of adventure and service, Betsi Cadwaladr died in 1860 and was buried in a pauper's grave.

Further Reading

Betsy Cadwaladyr: A Balaclava Nurse: An Autobiography of Elizabeth Davis (1857) was reprinted by Honno Classics in 1987 and 2007 with a useful introduction from Deirdre Beddoe and is your most important resource for her life.

Chapter 14

The Many Wars of Florence Nightingale

Though we think of her as the Lady With the Lamp, tirelessly patrolling the sick wards of the Crimean War offering solace and healing to soldiers who had been essentially left to die, Florence Nightingale's arguably greatest contributions came from a period in her life when illness prevented her from leaving the four walls of her modest living space. By then the most famous woman in England next to Queen Victoria herself, she could have enjoyed a life of ease and acclaim, but opted instead to drive herself, and those around her, at a health-ruining pace to compile statistics, gather reports and write up plans of action, in a grand and constantly frustrated attempt to remake the laws for how humans treat their sick.

In fact, no emotion winds its way through the tale of Nightingale's life with anything like the same evil persistence as Frustration. Frustration with herself, with her family, with her allies, with her enemies, with bureaucracy, with women generally and high-born women particularly, with prime ministers and viceroys – nobody was ever quite up to scratch in Florence Nightingale's precise yet merciless estimation, and anything short of total victory had to be reckoned as abject failure.

The origin of Nightingale's iron streak is difficult to pinpoint, born more out of opposition to her upbringing than evolving therefrom. Her father was an affable, scholarly gentleman whose ideal was to be left alone to ponder metaphysics, while her mother and sister focused upon making their home a hub of effervescent social activity. Florence played the role of Elizabeth Bennet in this divided household, studying foreign languages, history and philosophy with her father, but not taking herself so seriously that she snubbed opportunities for fun (in particular a good dance) that came her way.

She could not stand, however, wasting time in the endless rounds of house calls and rumour-mongering letters that were the expected mainstays of her station in life, and often hoped for some occupation beyond the rigidly organised leisure that obsessed her mother and sister. Then, in February 1837, she received what she believed to be a direct message from God, a verbal communication calling her to serve him. For a decade and a half, that moment ruined her life, making her feel suicidal levels of shame for doing anything that did not in some way measure up to a divine level of importance and merit. Her notes from the time, scribbled on pieces of paper she had at hand, are those of a young woman berating herself as a failure, a broken vessel unable to satisfy the needs of her family or of her divine calling, useless to all, and perhaps better off dead.

Nightingale was prone to episodes of prolonged intense daydreaming that were the shameful agony of her existence. In the middle of conversations, for long hours over the course of a day, she would snap into a world of intense fancy that she did not have the desire or will to leave, so uninspiring were the choices around her in reality. Were she born today, she would probably consider the God's Command episode as psychologically an extension of her intense compulsion to daydream, but as it was the nineteenth century, she considered it an actual physical intervention by a 3,000-year-old mythological character come to offer insistent, if vague, career advice, and that belief dominated her mental state for the coming difficult years.

She felt she *must* find some cause to prove herself in, while her family felt that it was simply rank ingratitude to hunger after anything more than the very comfortable life they provided for her. When, in 1845, she revealed to her family that she believed nursing was where her destiny lay, her mother and sister wailed, berating her for being so selfish as to destroy the family reputation with such a lowly choice of profession. Any subsequent mention of a desire to even visit a nursing institution to see what went on there inspired renewed outbursts, and it was not until 1851, fourteen hard, self-flagellating years after her original divine calling, that she was able to take the first practical step in what was to be her life's work.

That was the year she was able to finally visit the Kaiserwerth Institution and observe the nursing practices there first hand. It was neither a terribly clean nor well-run institution, but the nurses there were of exemplary character and devotion, a decided contrast to the reputation that nurses had earned in Europe as being low class, promiscuous drunkards who, likely as not, doubled as prostitutes in their spare time. Nightingale's mission, as it emerged in the coming years, was to recreate British nursing with the high tone of Kaiserwerth, but married to the scientific insights – as gained through rigorous statistical analysis – of modern scientific practice.

Between such scattered incidents of up-close observation and her systematic reading of the available nursing literature, Nightingale had gained a reputation in certain circles as somebody with a rare command of the practical needs of a medical institution; it was in this capacity that she was called in 1853 to serve as superintendent for the gloriously named Institution for the Care of Sick Gentlewomen in Distressed Circumstances. The Institution thought they were hiring a gifted fellow high-class socialite who would put time in here and there, as the spirit took her. What they got was a dynamo of reform, who saw at an instant what must be done, and what must be procured to do it, and relentlessly prodded all concerned until it was accomplished.

She was, it turned out to the surprise of all, a born administrator, with the ability to translate large-scale needs into the series of small-scale actions necessary to meet them. This reputation, along with her considerable knowledge of the nursing profession, lead to the offer from her friend Sidney Herbert, the Secretary at War, to lead a group of nurses to Scutari to see what might be done to improve the lot of those wounded in action while carrying out the variously misguided and undersupplied actions collectively known as the Crimean War.

She agreed, and on 5 November 1854, she and her nurses set foot in the infamous Barrack Hospital of Scutari, where they were met with open hostility by the doctors in attendance, who determined that they would not be put to use in lessening the suffering of the men strewn throughout the rooms and corridors, there to die in soiled and infested garments by the hundreds and thousands. Three roads lay open to Nightingale: to read the room and leave; to force her way past the doctors and put her nurses to work over their will and desires; or to sit at Scutari and wait until they came to her. Many of the nurses under her, motivated by the clear suffering of the men, wanted her to take the second option, but Nightingale knew instinctively that any attempt to force themselves upon the doctors' domain would breed nothing but resentment that would make eventual collaboration impossible.

She decided to wait, employing her nurses in whatever tasks had not explicitly been forbidden them by the doctors, and determining the true state of the hospital's arcane provisioning system. Sooner or later, she felt, the doctors would have to come to her, and the hospital's functioning would be helped by the spirit of cooperation, instead of hindered by one of resentment. Eventually, of course, they did seek her out, when the sheer scale of the human disaster in the Crimea overwhelmed the capacity of the Barrack Hospital to even remotely handle. Huge vats of diarrhoeal faeces lay open in the halls as the only means of relief since the rudimentary lavatory system had long since clogged and ceased to function. Vermin ran rampant through the halls. The walls sweated moisture and grew mould. Food was insufficient and irregular. Fresh clothing and bedding were available in the storehouses, but because of the British requisition system, none of it had been distributed in the hospital, so men died in the urine-and-faeces-stained clothes in which they had left the warfront weeks before.

Into this maelstrom of unnecessary death and disease strode Florence Nightingale. Her efforts were hampered on all sides: by the Catholic nuns among her nurses who refused to recognise her authority; by the requisitions officers who declined to distribute warehouses' worth of goods for fear of overstepping their minutely defined authority; and by administrators who sought to hide their misconduct by smearing her name back home. And yet, by dint of an unbreakable will that surprised even herself, she succeeded in pushing through reforms. Out of her own funds, she purchased goods and distributed them on her own authority to the wounded. The lavatories were flushed and cleaned. New diets were created for the various needs of her patients, and a system erected to see to its equitable distribution. A new hospital wing was built, again on her authority, that saved untold lives in the surges of wounded and ill soldiers that followed. Windows were opened, floors were scrubbed, clothes and sheets were changed and cleaned.

Having set reform at the Barrack Hospital in Scutari on its way, Nightingale's next task was to put the other military hospitals connected to the Crimean conflict in order. These were the hospitals where the nurses who had chaffed under her approach to nursing had fled, in particular the rebellious Catholic contingent under Mother Bridgeman. The hospitals under the care of these rogue nurses were in a sad state, desperately needing organisation, but Nightingale's original commission was as superintendent of the Female Nursing Establishment of the English General Hospitals in Turkey, a fact which administrators used to argue that she had no authority over nurses in Crimean hospitals that did not happen to be *in* Turkey.

As she was fighting to gain the authority to do the things that desperately needed to be done in the face of a system which desperately wanted its towering deficiencies to remain hidden, Florence Nightingale fell deathly ill with a case of Crimean fever, and for two weeks her death was believed to be imminent. She survived, but her attempts to institute meaningful reform in the non-Turkish military hospitals foundered on bureaucratic inertia and religious rebellion until her position as general superintendent of the nurses of all military hospitals was confirmed in 1856, thereby giving her, at last, the clear authority she needed to bring the other Crimean hospitals in line with her Scutari reforms.

That cable, however, reached her in March, just a month before the end of the war, and four months before the departure of the last patient from the Scutari hospital. She was given authority, in other words, at almost the exact moment when the only thing to do with that authority was to oversee the dismantling of the system it was meant to have created. Nightingale returned home in late July 1856, a hero in a conflict desperately lacking them. She was so unreservedly beloved that she could have bent her public adulation to the task of accomplishing medical reform by leading a broad-based popular movement, but again she stuck to her belief that the way to achieve reform was to work within the system. And so began the second, and I would say possibly even more heroic, stage of Nightingale's public career.

These years and decades lack the tragic-romantic imagery of her Crimean work, but in terms of persistent and largely thankless self-sacrifice, there are few things in the annals of all history to match her efforts of the 1850s, 1860s, and 1870s. Her physical health had been ruined by her time in the Crimea so that, as the years wore on, she was reduced entirely to a life lived between the walls of her various living spaces, sitting in bed with nothing but her ceaselessly scratching pen and steady flow of selected visitors to connect her with the outside world. She became enamoured of the raw power of statistical analysis to present arguments concisely and forcefully, and much of her life was engaged in collecting, from hospitals the world over, as much raw data as they could provide, and then painstakingly condensing that data into visual statistical representations, the use of which she pioneered, which were the ancestors of the charts and graphs we are exposed to in every news cycle as a matter of course today.

She made herself the century's indispensable expert on hospital design and medical practice, whose encyclopaedic command of how each reform translated, in verifiable numerical terms, into lowered mortality and illness rates, won over even the most sceptical of administrators sent to interview her. She was asked to serve on a Royal Commission investigating the health of the army, a task to which she applied all her organisational genius and apparently boundless inner energy. Her problem was, of course, her gender, which meant that, though she was the central hub of information and reform policy, she needed to rely on others to attempt to implement that policy in government, others whose efforts could never attain the heights of her expectations.

And yet, the astounding fact is that, in spite of expending so much effort time and again in amassing data and writing lengthy proposals of reform which, time and again, disappeared down the gullet of British bureaucracy, never to be seen again, she kept trying. When a scandal broke about the health system in India, she made it her business to send out detailed questionnaires to every medical hospital in the Raj as the first step in a massive effort to determine the relevant health statistics of the situation, making herself, a person who had never set foot in India, *the* world expert on Indian medical practices and their shortcomings. She proposed a radical overhaul not only of how the British ran their hospitals in India but of how the country was administered as a whole, encouraging the development of irrigation as a first step in improving the overall health of the land – the good effects of which would ripple through to the state of the hospitals. Prospective viceroys came to her dwelling to sit by her bed and receive their education about the land they were due to administer, and yet, in spite of all the oaths to do better, each regime largely failed to implement the most basic of her ideas, to the detriment of millions.

Faced with frustration and vexation in her attempts to get the overall health system of the empire to reform its worst practices, Nightingale met with better success in her secondary mission: the elevation of the nursing profession. In 1860, she established the Nightingale Training School (still in operation) at St Thomas's Hospital as an experiment in producing nurses of the calibre she had so desperately needed, but so rarely possessed, in the Crimea. Prospective nurses at the school were not only to be trained using the most modern methods but minutely observed to ensure that their character would bring credit to the nursing profession. They were even instructed to keep a diary which was regularly submitted to Nightingale and the school authorities for review in order to ascertain the purity of their minds and instincts.

The institution was a success, but Nightingale would forever lament, to anybody who might care to listen, the lack of qualified applicants, a fact which lay at the heart of her rather pessimistic evaluation of women as a gender. She bemoaned the fact that her school had so many requests for qualified nurses coming in from all corners of the country but so few people to send out to those assignments because so few qualified individuals had applied to the school. Growing up surrounded by women who floated in seas of free time that could be profitably spent in service of others, it baffled Nightingale that only a small number would take the opportunity represented by her school to do some real good. Nevertheless, the success of her students in overseeing their own hospital nursing staffs, combined with the mythic status of her time as the Lady With the Lamp, resulted in a definite shift in the perception of nurses over the course of the late nineteenth century. It drove the professionalisation of the career, albeit in directions Nightingale did not always support.

In the last decade of her life, following years of frustration in which she had to tend to her family's failing health while relinquishing the active reform that sustained her, she slipped at last into a more equitable appreciation of what she had accomplished in her time. Instead of declaring that she had failed in everything she had ever attempted because she had not obtained total victory on every point, she came to see the value of the partial steps that had been taken, and the worth of the momentum she had begun. Her last few years saw her sink into increasing blindness but also a peaceful seeming senility, much as her mother had at her life's end, not understanding entirely where she was or what was being said to her, but enjoying the pleasures of the day as they arrived until finally, on 13 August 1910, Florence Nightingale fell asleep, never to awake.

Further Reading

Many people's first in-depth experience of Florence Nightingale's life probably came in the form of Lytton Strachey's devastating portrait in *Eminent Victorians* (1918) which, while admiring her good traits, primarily delighted in her less heroic ones, such as her various metaphysical obsessions. It is certainly a fun read because Lytton Strachey is one of history's most gifted biographical stylists, but if you want something of more balance, I would go for Cecil Woodham-Smith's 1951 biography, which contains maybe my favourite first line of any Women in Science book. Of course, you might want something written *this* century in which case Mark Bostridge's 2008 book is probably what you are looking for.

Chapter 15

From the Underground Railroad to the Plantations of Santo Domingo

The Doctor's Journey of Sarah Loguen Fraser

In 1849, Elizabeth Blackwell became the first woman to earn a medical degree in the United States; within half a century 7,000 American women had followed her example. Twelve years prior to that, in 1837, James McCune Smith became the first black American male to earn such a degree (though he had to travel to the University of Glasgow to do so), and by 1920 there were nearly 4,000 practising black physicians in the United States. Yet while the turn of the twentieth century saw both women and black persons gradually but definitively entering the medical profession, the intersection of those two groups, comprised of black women physicians, lagged far behind the trends of its two constituent classes, with only sixty-five registered practitioners by the 1920s.

Black women who wanted to pursue a medical career had to face a persistent dual prejudice – denigrated for their gender and dismissed for their race – lacking institutions to help them along in their very particular life's course; prospective black women medical students required either unusually favourable social positions or unusually deep reserves of resolve to see their way through the early stages of their medical training. Eliza Anna Grier (?–1902), for example, was a former slave who took seven years to complete her medical courses at Fisk University because for every year she studied she had to take a year off to work to earn enough money for the next year of education. Grier's iron will to be educated was undeniably phenomenal, but most black women who earned degrees in the late nineteenth century did so because they came from relatively prosperous and prominent families who had the social connections and financial wherewithal to see them through their university years.

There are dozens of these stories to be told, and everybody has a different vote for which should be held up as the gold standard archetype, but few stories contain as many diverse elements of late nineteenth-century American culture as that of Sarah Loguen Fraser (1850–1933). Born in the year of the Compromise of 1850 which included the Fugitive Slave Act that enflamed abolitionist sentiment in the North and brought the nation one step closer to Civil War, Loguen (referred to as Logan in some sources) would be directly involved with abolitionist causes for the full span of her childhood. Her father, Reverend Jermain Loguen, was a key member of the Underground Railroad, and his Syracuse home was a major hub of its operations.

Sarah's youth was filled with the regular arrival of new individuals desperately seeking freedom, their speech struggling to convey the inhumanity of the world they had escaped. Over 1,500 people owed their freedom in part to Reverend Loguen, and so prominent was his part in the aid of runaway slaves that he himself had to flee to Canada for some time to avoid arrest on account of his role in the Jerry Rescue of 1851, which publicly rescued a fugitive slave who had been arrested under the provisions of the 1850 Act.

Raised in a household that counted Frederick Douglass and Gerrit Smith as particular friends, and Harriet Tubman as a close acquaintance, and by a mother who had graduated from the Oneida Institute and who emphasised to all her eight children the importance of working for the benefit of humanity, Sarah had everything that one could hope for in terms of ready-to-hand mentoring and inspiration. Both her parents were keenly aware of the value of education (they were central figures in establishing a series of schools in Syracuse to further black education), and ensured that she began attending school at the age of 5 and learning German, the language in which the most modern advances in chemical and medical knowledge were being promulgated in the late nineteenth century.

Loguen's early years were filled with learning, but also loss. An older sister died when she was 5, followed by her mother when she was 17, and then her father when she was 22. Up to that point, her life had been defined by service in her father's cause, particularly after the death of her mother and the marriage of her sister left her as the primary household organiser for a series of years. In 1873, however, she was at a railroad station when she saw a boy struck by a large farm wagon and crushed. She was filled with the hopelessness of watching a young life ebb away while she could do nothing to aid or soothe him. She resolved that: 'I will never see a human being in need and not be able to help.'

She spoke with a friend of the family, Dr Michael Benedict, a military doctor who had served in the Civil War, and who happened to board her train sometime after her witnessing of the accident. He had long championed women's medical education, and after ascertaining the depth of Loguen's commitment, agreed to tutor her in what she would need to enter a medical programme. She was admitted to Syracuse University's newly launched medical school (where Benedict was a faculty member) in 1873 and had graduated by 1876, becoming the fourth black woman in the United States to obtain a medical degree (behind Rebecca Lee (1864), Rebecca Cole (1867), and Susan Steward (1870)).

On the strength of a recommendation from the always encouraging Dr Benedict, Loguen was offered an internship at the Women's Hospital of Philadelphia, where she came immediately into conflict with a Dr Logue whose grandfather had owned Loguen's grandmother and father, and was in fact her father's father. Dr Logue did not much take to working with somebody whose very existence was a sign of her own family's dark past, and she left the hospital rather than face up to the weight of that inheritance. Loguen, however, stayed on and undertook the important work of venturing into the city's tenements and ministering to their various medical needs.

In 1878, she was invited to fill a six-month absence at the already legendary New England Hospital for Women and Children founded in Boston in 1862 by Marie Zakrzewska. There were no race barriers at the New England Hospital, which not only took on promising doctors like Loguen, but also established a nursing school which was the first in the nation to admit and graduate black nursing students.

Her time in Philadelphia and Boston gave Loguen the experience she needed to establish her own practice, which she did in Washington DC in 1879, building up a substantial client base on the strength of her skills and her family's good name, putting in long hours in the face of a plethora of diseases, one of which, malaria, she contracted in 1881. While recovering from this illness, she received a proposal of marriage from a wealthy pharmacist and plantation owner from Santo Domingo, Charles Fraser, who Loguen knew as a friend of Frederick Douglass's son. Douglass vouched for his character, and the prospect of a life of financial independence in a new setting with a man who would encourage her medical career was certainly enticing, and in 1882 the couple married.

Loguen relocated to Puerto Plata in Santo Domingo, where Fraser's flourishing businesses allowed her the social status and financial resources to start her practice in a land that had never known a female physician before. The fourth black woman MD in America, she was the first woman physician ever to practise in Santo Domingo, and upon announcing her services, she was inundated with clients seeking an alternative to the two lone other doctors serving in Puerto Plata. She had her first and only child in 1883, to whom we are indebted for most of our knowledge of Loguen's career, and in 1884 moved to a new house that had custom-built rooms for her flourishing practice.

For a beautiful decade, Loguen had all the satisfying work and respect that she could desire. Then, in 1894, Charles Fraser died from a stroke, and the maintenance of his plantation and running of his pharmacy fell suddenly on the shoulders of someone either too deep in grieving or too uninspired by the demands of business to carry either on. She sold the plantation in 1895, the pharmacy in 1897, and in 1901 moved back to Syracuse while Santo Domingo slipped into governmental chaos.

For a number of years, she wandered between different family members, caring for each in turn as they succumbed to disease and old age, until in 1908 she decided to become a resident physician at an industrial boys' school. If she was hoping to regain some of the challenge and respect of her Santo Domingo years, she was soon disabused of that notion. The school treated her as little more than a servant and maid in spite of her medical degree. The woman who had once been the medical treasure of an island was found by her nephew and daughter ironing, washing and cooking for the school's students.

She did escape that position thanks to her relatives, who railroaded over the school's attempts to say that she was legally bound to remain in her position until her death, but she never returned to the profession that had brought her so much satisfaction in younger days. She died in 1933 at the age of 83 at the home of her daughter, who took great comfort in the fact that her mother expired during the day, surrounded by the light of the sun.

Further Reading

Sarah Loguen Fraser's daughter Gregoria Fraser Goins wrote our primary source for Loguen's life, *Underground Railroad Princess: Sarah Loguen Fraser, MD*, which has, for who can say what possible reason, not yet been published. As such, we are left to hear about her life from people who have had access to that manuscript and shared its contents in one form or another with the world. *'Send Us a Lady Physician' Women Doctors in America: 1835–1920* is a wonderful resource from 1985 which features a chapter on the history of black women physicians in the late nineteenth and early twentieth centuries, but less than a paragraph on Loguen. For a more complete perspective, *Three Nineteenth-Century Women Doctors: Elizabeth Blackwell, Mary Walker and Sarah Loguen Fraser* (2007) has a very nice chapter by Susan Keeter, who as an artist is also responsible for one of the most famous representations of Loguen.

Chapter 16

Too Bright

Dr Anandibai Joshee, India's First Woman Medical Doctor

At 9 years old, a girl named Yamuna Joshee was married to her tutor, a man twenty years her senior, who thereupon changed her first name to Anandibai.

At 14, she gave birth to, and lost, her only child.

At 21, she became the world's first Indian woman to receive a medical degree.

Less than a year later, she was dead.

There is nothing small in the tale of Dr Joshee (1865–1887), a woman who planted herself squarely against the prejudices of two civilisations in pursuit of her country's good. Mocked in the streets of India for her dedication to medical study, she came to America only to find her Hindu customs and culture the object of smug, if well-meaning, drawing-room condescension. She battled cultural inertia, bureaucratic torpor and religious prejudice all while simultaneously fighting against the consumption that would ultimately take her life, finding time somewhere in the middle of all that to study and practise medicine.

She had been marked for greatness almost since she could talk. While a young girl, she had a dream about a man in curious armour who told her that she was meant to walk in his footsteps. After telling her father about her dream, he took her to the family's sacred records of ancestry, which she had never seen before, and asked if anybody looked familiar. Page after page went by, going deeper and deeper into the past, until finally the girl recognised the man from her dreams: the heroic founder of the family line. Taking Yamuna's dream as a direct communication from their ancestor, her father resolved to provide her with anything she needed to achieve her destiny.

A major component of that support came in the form of education. A distant relation by the name of Gopal Joshee was engaged to teach her Sanskrit and whatever else he happened to know. He was a widower, some twenty years her senior, and, when it came time for him to leave to take up a postmaster position elsewhere, she was disconsolate over the loss of her teacher. It was decided the best thing to do would be for the two to get married so that she could travel with him to his new post. She was 8 years old, and the marriage ceremony was carried out on her ninth birthday. As was tradition, the groom gave his bride a new name – no longer Yamuna, the child bride was now Anandibai, which translates as 'Joy of My Heart'.

She was intelligent and industrious, qualities which brought on the mockery of the more conservative elements of late nineteenth-century Indian society. The girl who was used to an intellectually supportive environment found herself insulted in the streets for failing in her duties as a high-caste Indian wife:

> Once it happened that I was obliged to stay in school for some time, and go twice a day for my meals to the house of a relation. Passers-by, whenever they saw me going, gathered round me. Some of them made fun, and were convulsed with laughter. Others, sitting respectably in their verandahs, made ridiculous remarks, and did not feel ashamed to throw pebbles at me. The shopkeepers and vendors spit at the sight of me, and made gestures too indecent to describe.

In spite of the mockery and abuse, she remained committed to her path of the mind, one which achieved new focus when she lost her first and only child shortly after birth. She was convinced that what her country most desperately needed was women in the medical profession, trained in the newest advances of Western medicine. She would go to America, learn all she could, and then bring that knowledge back to India to train more doctors and thereby raise the standard of women's health in her country.

No sooner did she announce her intention than protests arose from all sides. Traditional elements of Indian society declared that, left alone in America, she would betray her traditions and beliefs. Christian missionary societies that could have eased her way to America balked when she said she would not convert to Christianity. To answer her detractors, she took the unprecedented step of announcing a public speech in which she would lay out what she intended to do, and why she desired to do it.

On 24 February 1883, a 17-year-old Indian girl stood up before her elders in a packed hall of sceptics and plain gawkers, and declared the contents of her mind and heart:

> You ask of me, why I should do what is not done by any of my sex? To this I can only say, that society has a right to our work as individuals.
>
> It is very difficult to decide the duties of individuals. It is enough that the good of one must be the good of all. If anything seems best for all mankind, each one of us must try to bring it about. So I am surprised to hear that I should not do this, because it has not been done by others. Our ancestors whose names have become immortal had no such notions in their heads … To desist from duty because we fear failure or suffering is not just. **We must try.** Never mind whether we are victors or victims. Manu has divided people into three classes. The meanest are those who never attempt anything for fear of failure. Those who begin, and are disheartened by the first obstacles, come next; but those who begin, and persevere through failure and obstacle, are those who win.

The confidence and wisdom of her speech were applauded, and it was widely published in the papers, attracting sponsors and well-wishers who ultimately smoothed her road to America. On 7 April she was on her way, the first unconverted high-caste Indian woman to leave India. Her destination was the Women's Medical College of Philadelphia, where she would have to squeeze her studies in between the duties of being An Attraction for the high society set.

An Indian student in America, she wore traditional clothing, ate only vegetarian fare, and maintained her religious and cultural practices, all of which was irresistible to a dinner party circuit seeking distraction amidst comfort. She was invited to parties, asked to sing her 'quaint' native songs, quizzed a hundred times over about her clothes, and treated to the sights and sounds of society matrons who considered her nose jewellery 'savage' but who enjoyed being Big Enough to overlook it in deference to her character. As her only significant English language biographer, Caroline Healey Dall, who was herself of the dinner party set, managed to say, 'The longer Anandibai lived in America the less she liked to wear her ornaments, or rather those ornaments which, like the ear-rings and the nose-ring, recalled a savage condition of society. [But] when *she* wore them, they did not offend me.'

According to Dall, Anandibai was quite happy to perform for her American hosts, cooking traditional meals for them, singing on demand, and wrapping them in exotic saris for soirees. How she actually felt, we cannot say, for the same blindness to her own cultural condescension that marks Dall's more unfortunate comments about the 'Hindu character' could well have prevented her from accurately seeing her class's attentions as sources of continuous embarrassment or imposition.

The true enemy, however, during Anandibai's three years in America, was not the often smug but consistently supportive superiority of her hosts, but her own body. She had suffered from headaches since her mid-teens, and came down with diphtheria on at least one occasion, but as her American sojourn lengthened, she noticed the headaches getting worse, followed by an ominous cough and shortness of breath that heralded the arrival of tuberculosis. The progress of the disease was not helped by her friends, who insisted that strenuous trips to different parts of the country were just the thing she needed to recover. Too polite to decline these offers, Anandibai wore herself out on these trips and parties, but managed to graduate at last in 1886. Shortly thereafter, she won an appointment as the physician-in-charge at the Female Ward of Albert Edward Hospital in Kolhapur, India.

India's first licensed woman doctor, lauded on three different continents for her success, had her dream in her grasp – an opportunity to apply her new knowledge in her home country. But it was not to be. After a rough passage back to India, during which her husband broke fundamental caste restrictions by attending on her day and night as her nurse, Anandibai was welcomed with acclaim and pride by the same people who had vilified her only four years earlier. In spite of the rapid deterioration of her condition, she insisted on returning to her home town, to visit once again the sites of her childhood. Her uncle put her up in the house where she was born, feeling a premonition that it would also be the house where she passed. On 26 February 1887, Anandibai Joshee died, not yet 22 years old, never having had the chance to put the skills she had worked so hard to acquire at the service of the people she hoped to save.

Her last words were, 'I have done all that I could.' And she had.

Further Reading

For years, the only real source of substance we had in English for Anandibai Joshee was Dall's 1888 biography, *The Life of Dr Anandibai Joshee, A Kinswoman of the Pundita Ramabai*. She spends more time talking about

Anandibai's clothes and society impressions than she does about her actual medical work, accuses Gopal of gross ingratitude whenever he speaks out against Imperial treatment of India, and drops lines every so often like, 'It is not learning, intellect, subtlety, or imagination that is wanting in the average Hindu; it is purity, faith and honesty.' To read her book is to see Anandibai through the gauze of a prejudice that is doubly dangerous in that it thinks itself enlightened, and so you come away with some general outlines, but never feel as though you have touched the real person. Fortunately, in 2020 Nandini Patwardhan published *Radical Spirits: India's First Woman Doctor and Her American Champions*, breaking the nearly century and a half drought of available material.

Chapter 17

A Healer at the Fringe of Civilisation

The Siberian Odyssey of Doctor Anna Bek

It is the early 1870s and we are heading into the mining town of Gornyi Zerentui, located in the mountainous Transbaikal region on the distant Siberian fringe of Imperial Russia. Here political prisoners are sent to work the mines for bare subsistence pay, overseen by the descendants of former political exiles, like the director of the mine whose house we are currently stepping into. It is filled with poor relations, doing their part to keep the household running as a way of earning their keep; our interest is not in them but in the nursery where we shall find the household nanny sleeping in a makeshift bed while next to her three children slumber on the floor, sweetly oblivious to the scurrying sounds of omnipresent cockroaches.

One of those sleeping children is Anna Nikolaevna (1869–1954) and what she can expect from her life here in a part of Europe as yet untouched by railway and indoor plumbing is a marriage to a mining engineer, the raising of ten or so children, and a slow descent deathward, all contained within a radius of perhaps 50 miles. But Anna, you see, has a *mind*, a phenomenal mind which will send her to the mightiest capitals of Europe, and all across the sweeping vastness of Imperial Russia.

It will also get her into a great deal of trouble, but for now she is the golden child, full of promise. Sitting underneath the dining room table while her older sisters have lessons in reading and writing, she seems to absorb the concepts immediately and naturally to the astonishment of all her family. Her sisters tell her repeatedly that she must ask their father to be allowed to go away to school in Irkutsk, some 950 miles away but still the closest school of any steady reputation, and one day, summoning all her courage, she does. And he, to the surprise of everyone, agrees.

Anna's life, first at Gornyi Zerentui then at the Gugda mine, was a carefree one before her departure for formal schooling in 1882. She learned new things, romped through nearby forests, gathered berries and burned tree stumps, without a thought for the next day. At the Institute for Noble

Girls in Irkutsk, however, her life took a sudden Dickensian turn as she was stuffed in a three-storey stone house with the barest minimum of food to eat and smothering restrictions on all activity. It was a place of little personal joy, but intellectually Anna flourished, given proper mental sustenance at last. She learned German and French and was soon top of her class, in which capacity she became the particular interest of the school's new director, Konstantin Frantsevich, who inspired her with the thought that knowledge was only any good if it could be employed in the active helping of other people.

Graduating with Highest Honours in 1888, she had reached the pinnacle of what might be expected for a woman in provincial Russia. She had heard rumours of Higher Women's Courses being offered in the imperial capital of St Petersburg, but that was 4,600 miles away, a month's journey under the best of available conditions, and besides the Women's Courses were reputed to be a wicked institution where women learned materialism and, gasp of gasps, atheism, as a result of their increased knowledge of the crude mechanisms of bodily functioning.

At first, Anna did not set her sights as high as St Petersburg but decided to settle down as a teacher of some sort in her home town and to do good in that fashion. To that end, she and some friends founded a small school, but upon the death of her mother she had the guilty thought that, if she had applied herself more, had stretched her brain and become a doctor, she might have been able to save her. When she read in one of her father's papers the announcement of a new school, the Women's Medical Institute, to be founded in St Petersburg with the tsar's own approval, she formed her plans in an instant to attend and began cramming the Greek and Latin that would be required for her entrance exam.

In 1894, without having previously written to the Institute to discover its present status, she and her brother set out for St Petersburg, stringing together a chain of horses-and-carts, precarious ferries, and finally railroad cars to cover the distance in a brisk thirty-one days, only to discover upon arrival that the Institute was not open, and would not be any time soon. The Higher Women's Courses were still running, however, and, impressed by Nikolaevna's Irkutsk transcripts, they accepted her immediately. Here, Nikolaevna was able to further her higher general education, but it was not the place to further one's medical knowledge and so she went to the city that had, for decades, been a refuge for women the world over seeking medical training: Paris.

Did she write ahead, to inquire about how likely it was that she would be accepted by a Paris medical university, before making the trip? You know enough at this point to know that the answer is *no* and, once again, the promising young student arrived in a city only to find that it did not have a place for her. It was 1895, an election year, and the government had decided to stand firm against the waves of foreigners who were taking up places at the university that ought to be going to Frenchmen.

Rejected by Paris, all was, however, not lost, for there were still the French provinces, which were eager to accept high-calibre students, and where a top-rate education could still be had. Nikolaevna ended up in Nancy, where she fell in instantly with a group of Russian-speaking women students who formed her intellectual entourage, supporting her emotionally and practically as she stormed ahead with a rigorous exam schedule. She achieved top marks again, but her score was later lowered by the administration so that a foreigner would not take first place on the exam rolls.

Her education was humming along when she heard that the Women's Medical Institute would finally be opening in 1897, at which point she dropped everything to return to her much-missed native soil and join the first class. The topics of her first years there were rehashings of material she had learned in Nancy, and this gave her time to get involved with the intellectual scene that late nineteenth-century St Petersburg had to offer. These were heady times to be a student in the imperial capital. Young intellectuals were looking away from tsarist autocracy to bold new ideas in governance, with socialism and communism forming the stuff of a thousand dinner conversations held nightly throughout the city.

Nikolaevna was a founding member of a Marxist discussion circle that met regularly to sing workers' songs and discuss different points of communist philosophy, and when the government began drafting students in Kiev for military service in 1901, she was one of the primary organisers of the Institute's general student strike against the government's actions. As a ringleader of the strike, she was targeted by the authorities, who decreed that she must leave the capital and go into exile for a period of one year, whereupon she returned home to serve out her time.

It was here, while in exile, that she met Evgeny Vladimirovich Bek, a conscientious, socially responsible and much-respected military doctor who had been given the job of roving Siberian physician after supporting the cause of the soldiers against the military administration in 1894. He and Anna were both committed medical practitioners who had been cast to the far reaches of the empire to keep their radical ideas far from the country's administrative centres. She respected and admired him greatly but was never head-over-heels in love with him, which might have been a problem had she not had enough run-ins as a student with romantic love to know that it ended in heartbreak and self-recriminations more often than not. He was a sturdy and admirable man who was interested in the same things she was and who did not blink at the idea of his potential wife continuing her medical education.

He would, in short, do fine.

They married in 1902 and the following year, after returning from her exile, Nikolaevna, now Bek, received her medical degree just in time for the couple to serve together as doctors in the military hospitals of the Russo-Japanese War (1904/5) where the full brunt of Russian administrative incompetence was impressed on them daily. By 1906, they were back in Siberia, in the small town of Aksha where Evgeny was doctor to the Cossack Host and Anna made strides in developing a community centre to act as a central location for dramatic productions, educational displays and book exchanges, in an overwhelmingly successful attempt to raise the self-awareness and educational standards for a region given primarily to drinking and fist-fights as its main avenue of entertainment.

Moving in 1912 to Chita, the capital of Transbaikal, she applied her knowledge of new trends in psychology (particularly the theories of Maria Montessori) to the development of a new school for the region that spawned the training of dozens of teachers and the rise of an engaged parent community who were astounded by what their children were capable of, given a systematic structure to operate within. As in Aksha, Anna and Evgeny divided their patient load between them, with Anna more often than not seeing to the needs of women patients who were uncomfortable with a male doctor, and who appreciated her competence and professionalism.

With the arrival of the First World War in 1914, however, life in Chita took a decided stumble towards chaos that would last the better part of a decade. Evgeny was detailed to serve in the Chita military hospital, where he once again advocated for the betterment of the soldiers' conditions (in this case an increase in their meagre rations) and once again was punished by the military administration with reassignment, this time to a Turkish typhus ward that was a virtual death sentence for a man of his age. In 1915, he duly caught typhus and died of it, leaving his wife to support their child in a region that was growing more unstable by the minute.

After the tsarist government fell in 1917, Chita became a crossroads in the subsequent Civil War which saw Soviet, tsarist and independent Cossack forces battling back and forth across the land, taking and losing the important political hub of Chita in turn while the citizens did the best they could to negotiate the constantly shifting ideological landscape. Anna was dedicated to reform and the championing of the workers' cause, but was not comfortable with openly siding exclusively with the Communist Party. She knew too many people who were doing good and useful work from all manner of different political perspectives to allow herself to take part in any movement that would force her to disavow the people whose goodness she believed in. She recalled in her memoirs, written some decades later,

> When one [member] of the Bolshevik Party … pointed out to me that by entering the party I could work on public education with greater success I was very confused; while I sympathised with the Bolsheviks, at the same time I knew that I was not suited to become a party member. One of my shortcomings was that I always evaluated people according to their moral qualities and not according to their political convictions. [transl. Anne Rassweiler].

This decision, to not openly declare herself a Bolshevik during the Civil War, would cause problems for her later, but she had made herself such a central part of the educational and medical system in Chita that she was retained with each change of ownership of the city, and only left in 1922 to be closer to her daughter, who lived at Irkutsk. Two decades had elapsed since Bek had been anywhere near the country's interior, and she was starting her sixth decade of life, but she was determined to remake herself as a university professor in an increasingly unpredictable and hostile political climate.

She took it as her life's work to espouse the benefits of reflexology and paedology, which at the time meant a holistic approach to child development which used anatomy, physiology and psychology together to evaluate and understand the different stages of human development. Rather than talking about abstract psyches or philosophically fashionable ideal concepts, she wanted to see how all the parts of the body work together to gradually create an adult being, and how we might use that knowledge of neural and motor development to create a better education system. While paedology was embraced at first by Soviet science as a solid, materially grounded counterbalance to Western medical mysticism, by 1936 it had fallen out of fashion, and Bek was forced from her position at the University of Tomsk in 1936 after refusing to disavow her belief in its scientific validity.

She found work in Novosibirsk for another seven years after that as a paediatrician and industrial trade school physician, but she would never again know the personal satisfaction she experienced in Chita as a medical practitioner and community organiser, nor the professional esteem she had experienced as an author of papers and researcher in the late 1920s when her paedological views were fashionable. She retired in 1944 to the role of grandmother, gifting the world one last treasure in the form of the memoirs she wrote in 1948 to tell her family a little bit about the remarkable life she had lived – starting on a floor in tsarist Siberia, and ending, quietly, one year after the fall of the Stalinism that had brought her academic career in the service of children to a premature end.

Further Reading

We would know none of this story without the work done by Anne D. Rassweiler in researching Bek's life, and translating and publishing her memoirs, which she did in *The Life of a Russian Woman Doctor: A Siberian Memoir, 1869–1954* (2004). It is an astounding document, and the book provides useful notes on the particular relation of Siberia to the rest of tsarist and Soviet Russia during this turbulent era. This is exactly the sort of research and publication we need more of – so many women wrote nothing of their lives, and of those who did, so many accounts remain obscure in the hands of families who do not entirely know what to do with them, and the more exchange there is between families possessing documents like this and academics who can bring them to the light of day, the better the world will be.

Chapter 18

Brief Portraits

The Nineteenth-Century Women's Medicine Renaissance

Harriot Kezia Hunt (1805–1875)

One of America's pioneers in the field of women doctoring, Hunt established her practice in 1835 after two years studying with Elizabeth and Richard Dixon Mott, who had treated her for tuberculosis. She carried on the Motts' principles, of using rest and herbal remedies to cure illnesses instead of more invasive or extreme practices, in her own practice. In 1847, she applied to Harvard Medical School, and was denied. She applied again after Elizabeth Blackwell received her degree in 1849, and was given permission to attend lectures, but a literal riot in 1850 by the student body caused the administration to rescind the invitation. She continued her practice, while also advocating for the abolition of slavery and instatement of women's suffrage.

Marie Durocher (1809–1893)

Born in Paris, Durocher moved with her family to Brazil when she was 8 years old. Generally considered to be the first woman doctor in Latin America, she took up medicine as a way to support her two children after the death of her husband. In 1834, she was the first woman to be granted a medical degree by the Medical School of Rio de Janeiro. She served as a physician for some six decades, drawing attention for her habit of dressing in practical men's clothes.

Ann Preston (1813–1872)

Preston was born to a Pennsylvania Quaker family of abolitionists who used their farm as a safe house for runaway slaves. Educationally progressive, Preston's family supported her attempt to receive a medical education, and in 1850 she was a student in the inaugural class of the Female Medical College of Pennsylvania, a Quaker institution aimed at the training of women medical professionals. She graduated the following year, and took up a post as professor of physiology and hygiene in 1853. In 1867, she became dean of the institution, now called the Woman's Medical College of Pennsylvania, and thereby also became the first woman dean of a modern medical institution. She continued in that capacity until her death in 1872.

Clara Harlowe Barton (1821–1912)

'Shame on you for sticking Clara Barton, the founder of the American Red Cross, a hero the world over, into a Brief Portrait!' Yes, I know. I am a bad person.

Clara Barton became a teacher at the age of 17 by way of her family's plan to help her overcome her extreme timidity. She continued at this profession until 1852 when she was asked to open a new free school in New Jersey. The school was a great success, and under Barton's stewardship grew to the point that it needed expanded facilities, at which point Barton was replaced by a man as principal, a woman being deemed unfit for managing a large institution such as the new school would become. She thereupon spent some time as a patent clerk until the American Civil War, when she began volunteering as a nurse to the soldiers returning from the war. By 1862, she had received permission to work on the front lines, where she soon received the nickname, 'Angel of the Battlefield'.

After the war, she travelled to Switzerland where she met Dr Louis Appia, a founder of the International Committee of the Red Cross who convinced her to open a branch in America, which soon became an epicentre of humanitarian response to crises the world over. In 1900, the American Red Cross was formally recognised by the US government, though Barton herself would be compelled to resign from her leadership role four years later, at the age of 83. Thereupon she established the National First Aid Society in 1905, which was later reabsorbed into the American Red Cross.

Emily Elizabeth Parsons (1824–1880)

Blind in one eye from a childhood accident, partially deaf from a childhood case of scarlet fever, and unable to stand for long periods because of an ankle injury, Emily Parsons seemed an unlikely person to become a wartime heroine, but with the arrival of the American Civil War, she felt she had no choice but to train herself as a nurse and offer her services to the Union army. By 1862, she had completed her training at Massachusetts General Hospital, and for two months that year she oversaw a medical ward at Fort Schuyler. She subsequently served on a hospital steamship that plied the Mississippi River in the wake of General Grant's army, tending to hundreds of invalided soldiers, and at the Benton Barracks Hospital, where she was in charge of operations that cared for approximately 2,000 men. Her memoirs were published in 1880, the year of her death.

Mary Amanda Dixon Jones (1828–1908)

A gynaecologist at the Women's Hospital of Brooklyn from 1882 to 1891, Jones was known for her surgical skills. In 1888, she performed the first hysterectomy in the United States, to treat uterine cancer, which resulted in the successful removal of a 17lb tumour. The following year, the newspaper *The Brooklyn Eagle* launched a series of investigations into the Women's Hospital, accusing Jones of forcing women to undergo her procedures. Those articles resulted in Jones being brought up on one count of murder, one count of manslaughter, and six counts of malpractice. She was ultimately found not guilty, but after losing the subsequent libel case against the *Eagle* she was compelled to close the Women's Hospital, and devoted her time to pathological studies in the vein of Mary Jacobi. She published over fifty medical papers over the course of her career.

Emeline Horton Cleveland (1829–1878)

Cleveland earned her MD from the Female Medical College of Pennsylvania in 1855, and after some time training in Paris and London, financed through the efforts of Ann Preston, became chief resident at the Woman's Hospital of Philadelphia in 1862, and in 1872 took over from Ann Preston as dean of the Women's Medical College of Philadelphia (formerly the aforementioned Female Medical College), a position she held until her poor health compelled her to step down in 1874. She established one of the world's first training facilities for nursing assistants, and, in the year of her death from tuberculosis, became a gynaecologist at the Pennsylvania Hospital Department for the Insane, which was one of the first instances in America of a woman joining the staff of a major American public hospital.

Marie Zakrzewska (1829–1902)

This is probably the one I feel the worst about relegating to a Brief Portrait because, by and large, that is how history has treated Marie Zakrzewska: as a figure mentioned briefly in the course of biographies about other people, such as Elizabeth Blackwell. She was, however, a central figure in the history of women's medical education and deserves far better than that. The daughter of Polish parents who fled Poland during the final partition of that country in order to avoid Russian rule, Zakrzewska was ultimately born in Berlin, where her mother took up work as a midwife when her father's military career failed to pay the family expenses. She accompanied her mother on her rounds, read all she could on medical practice, and applied at the age of 19 to join the Royal Charité Hospital in Berlin, which was an official governmental midwife school. Rejected on account of her young age, she applied again the following year, was rejected again, and then reapplied the *next* year, at which point the administration bowed before the might of her persistence and admitted her, where she became one of the institution's star students.

Graduating in 1851, she set out with her sister in 1853 for New York, where just four years previously Elizabeth Blackwell had earned her famous medical degree. America, however, was not so inviting to a young woman medical practitioner as she had hoped, and she and her sister were compelled to sell embroidered goods to make ends meet. Fortunately, one year later Marie met Elizabeth Blackwell at last, and was offered a position at Blackwell's Tompkins Square dispensary. Together with Emily and Elizabeth Blackwell, Zakrzewska was a founding figure of the subsequent New York Infirmary for Indigent Women and Children, where she regularly put in eighteen-hour days. In 1859, she moved to Boston, where she conceived the idea of founding a new institution which would give women doctors a chance to practise medicine that was denied them by most of the country's major hospitals. In 1862, she founded the New England Hospital for Women and Children, which aimed to give care to all who needed it, regardless of race or ability to pay, and which continues its existence to this day as the Dimock Community Health Center. The hospital also boasted the first American training school for nurses, which in 1879 graduated the first accredited black nurse, Mary Mahoney.

Rebecca Lee (née Davis) Crumpler (1831–1895)

Rebecca Crumpler was the first black woman to earn a medical degree in the United States, in 1864. She had begun her medical career as a nurse in 1855, following in the footsteps of her aunt, who was her community's go-to medical professional. In 1860, she applied and was accepted to the New England Female Medical College, which had been founded some twelve years earlier by Samuel Gregory for the purpose of giving women the medical knowledge needed to become certified midwives. After her historic graduation in 1864, she worked in Boston until the close of the Civil War. She then devoted herself to the work of the Freedmen's Bureau, the governmental department tasked with the monumental job of reuniting slave families, creating educational facilities for former slaves and their children, distributing food and land, and attending to the medical and political needs of the South's black population. Crumpler's work focused on providing medical care for black patients who were being systematically refused service by the white medical establishment.

In 1883, she wrote *A Book of Medical Discourses*, a work summarising the medical wisdom for women and children she had stored up over three decades as a nurse and doctor.

Emily Howard (née Jennings) Stowe (1831–1903)

Generally considered the first woman to professionally practise medicine in Canada, Howe was a teacher until her husband contracted tuberculosis, which renewed her interest in medicine and herbal treatments. She applied to the Toronto School of Medicine in 1865, and was summarily rejected on account of her gender. She then applied to the New York Medical College and Hospital for Women, which had been founded just two years previously by the physician and activist Clemence Lozier. She graduated in 1867 and returned to Toronto to open her private practice. Because she possessed a foreign licence, however, she was not permitted to obtain a Canadian medical licence until she took a series of required courses, which the University of Toronto refused to allow her to do. In 1871 she was given permission to attend classes at the Toronto School of Medicine, but she left before taking her final exams in protest at the behaviour of the male faculty and students. In 1880, she was finally given a medical licence from the College of Physicians and Surgeons of Ontario, making her the second woman in Canada to have a medical licence, behind Jennie Kidd Trout (1841–1921).

Chloe A. Buckel (1833–1912)

Buckel's life was cut from the purest of nineteenth-century cloth – her parents died before she was 1, then her grandparents before she was 4, resulting in her finally being placed in the hands of a pair of authoritarian aunts. She started teaching at the age of 14, and saved up her money to pay for a medical education. Using her slim savings, she attended the Woman's Medical College of Pennsylvania, and in 1858 studied under Marie Zakrzewska at the New York Infirmary for Indigent Women and Children. During the Civil War, she was responsible for the erection of six field hospitals and was one of a group of professionals appointed by Dorothea Dix to select prospective army nurses. In 1866, she rejoined Zakrzewska, now at the New England Hospital for Women and Children, where she was ultimately appointed as attending surgeon. With the decline of her health, however, she resigned from that high-stress position and set up a private practice in Oakland, California.

Lucy Ellen Sewall (1837–1890)

Lucy Sewall is another of those key figures who shows up at important moments during the nineteenth-century struggle for women's medical education who has yet to receive the full-volume treatment she deserves. A graduate of the New England Female Medical College in 1862, she joined Marie Zakrzewska's New England Hospital for Women and Children in 1864 as a staff physician, in which capacity she met and inspired Sophia Jex-Blake to become a doctor on the latter's tour of America. In addition to her official duties at the hospital, she seems to have had the unofficial duty of acting as the communications nexus and voice of reason connecting the various American and British medical pioneers who were all pulling in their own very different directions. In 1881, she attempted unsuccessfully to compel Harvard to open its doors to women (which it would not do until 1945).

Emilie Lehmus (1841–1932)

A pioneer for women's medical practice in Germany, Emilie Lehmus attended the University of Zurich, which had been offering medical degrees to women since 1864. There she met fellow German student Franziska Tiburtius (see below). She received her doctorate in 1870, and moved to Berlin, where she and Tiburtius established a clinic for women and children in 1877, and then a larger polyclinic (the first of its kind in Berlin) in 1881; it offered free treatment for poor women, and, like Zakrzewska's New England Hospital, gave women doctors crucial experience in their craft. Illness compelled Lehmus to give up her practice in 1900.

Varvara Aleksandrovna Kashevarova-Rudneva (1842–1899)

Varvara Rudneva was orphaned at an early age, and spent most of her childhood being kicked around between variously abusive foster families until she took her destiny in her own hands and fled to St Petersburg, where she married Nikolai Stepanovich Kashevarov, who had promised he would allow her to continue her studies, and whom she promptly left when he failed to keep his word. In 1862, she applied to the Princess Elena Pavlovna Lying-In-Home's midwife course, and finished the two-year curriculum in eight months. She then obtained a position as a midwife to a group of Muslim Bashkir troops in Orenburg. Religious restrictions meant that their wives could not be seen by male doctors, and the governor of Orenburg gave Rudneva a stipend to attend to them. He then supported her attempt to obtain a full medical degree at the Medical Surgical Academy, where she gained admittance because she was a woman seeking to tend to patients who were religiously prevented from seeking male treatment. By 1869, she had passed her preliminary examinations but withdrew her request to defend her dissertation in 1873 when the opposition it aroused threatened a new experimental programme to open medical education to women. It was not until 1878 that she was finally permitted to defend her thesis, on the early signs of uterine cancer, and received her medical doctorate, becoming only the second woman in Russia to earn that degree. Antisemitism combined with misogyny, however, to prevent her from obtaining a fixed and steady position commensurate with her skills.

Nadezhda Prokof'evna Suslova (1843–1918)

Nadezhda Suslova was both a revolutionary author and a revolutionary physician. During the early 1860s, she wrote a series of modern short stories that attracted the attention of the Imperial police, as did her joining of the covert revolutionary society, Land and Liberty. She was nevertheless allowed to attend the Imperial Military Medical Academy until women were banned from universities in Russia in 1865 (with the very occasional exception, as in the case of Varvara Rudneva, see above). She continued her education in Switzerland and Germany, earning her doctorate from

Graz Medical University in 1867, and then passing a special examination to validate that degree in Russia in 1868 – making her the first woman to receive a medical degree in Russia. Her subsequent practice in St Petersburg and Nizhny-Novgorod centred on diseases arising as the result of urban conditions, and on offering treatment to the Tatar community, who were often unable to pay for medical service.

Franziska Tiburtius (1843–1927)

Encouraged by her sister-in-law, Germany's first certified woman dentist, to study medicine after six years spent as a governess, Tiburtius took the same route as Emilie Lehmus (see above) and travelled to the University of Zurich, where she received her degree in 1876 and moved to Berlin, where she and Lehmus established their women's clinic in 1877 and polyclinic in 1881. In 1923 she published her memoirs.

Dame Mary Ann Dacomb (née Bird) Scharlieb (1845–1930)

Senior surgeon at the London School of Medicine for Women (founded by Sophia Jex-Blake and Elizabeth Garrett Anderson) from 1889 to 1902, Scharlieb began her medical career after moving with her husband to Madras and witnessing the state of gynaecological care in India. She studied midwifery and then entered Madras Medical College in 1875, one of the earliest women to attend that institution. Returning to England in 1878, she gained admittance to the London School of Medicine for Women – against Elizabeth Anderson's better judgment (she considered Scharlieb to be too frail for the rigours of the medical profession). She graduated in 1882, and in 1883 returned to India for four years to lecture at the Madras Medical College on topics related to gynaecology and midwifery. In 1888, she earned her MD in London, and the following year took over Elizabeth Garrett Anderson's post as chief surgeon at the London School. She retired from her various public posts in 1909.

Elsie (née Maude) Inglis (1846–1917)

Born in India, Elsie Inglis returned to her family's native Edinburgh at a young age, and in 1887 she was one of the first students to attend Sophia

Jex-Blake's Edinburgh School of Medicine for Women. She soon bristled under Jex-Blake's leadership style, however, and led an exodus from the school that resulted in the creation of the rival Edinburgh College of Medicine for Women, which ultimately put Jex-Blake's college out of business. Receiving medical licences from three different institutions in 1892, Inglis spent some time at Elizabeth Garrett Anderson's New Hospital for Women before returning to Edinburgh to found a new maternity hospital with Jessie MacLaren MacGregor. During the First World War, she organised the Scottish Women's Hospitals (SWH) for Foreign Service which provided fourteen fully equipped medical units and a staff of a thousand women that served throughout Europe. Inglis shipped out with the Serbian branch of the SWH, and was captured by the Central Powers in 1915 as she tried to organise the repatriation of wounded soldiers who had been left behind by the retreating Allies. Released in 1916, she joined the SWH team operating out of Odessa, but by 1917 her health had grown so poor that she was compelled to return to Britain, where she died of bowel cancer the day after setting foot back on British soil.

Anna Elizabeth Broomall (1847–1931)

A product of the Woman's Medical College of Pennsylvania, where she received her degree in 1868, and the Pennsylvania Hospital, where she earned her MD in 1871, Broomall went on to become the chief resident physician at the Woman's Medical College in Pennsylvania from 1875 to 1883, and assumed the chair of the obstetrics department at the Woman's Medical College in 1879 upon the death of Emeline Horton Cleveland. In 1888, she established an out-practice clinic in Philadelphia, where students of the college were assigned cases in pre- and post-natal care in the community. She retired in 1903.

Clara Marshall (1847–1931)

Marshall was the fourth dean of the Woman's College of Philadelphia, succeeding Rachel Bodley in 1888. She had previously attended the college as a student, where she was taught by a Who's Who list of American medical women – Ann Preston, Emeline Cleveland and Rachel Bodley. As dean, she oversaw the modernisation of the college, expanding the curriculum from a three-year to a four-year programme, establishing a bacteriology professorship, and initiating the construction of the Pavilion Hospital on campus in 1904. She retired as dean in 1917.

Anna Shabanova (1848–1932)

Shabanova was one of the early beneficiaries of Varvara Rudneva's decision to hold off on submitting her doctoral dissertation until 1878. Shabanova had returned to St Petersburg from her studies in Helsinki when the authorities announced in 1873 the beginning of their experiment of allowing women to attend university courses at the Women's Medical Courses in St Petersburg. She received her degree in 1878, and embarked on a career centred around the improvement of Russian paediatric medicine, including the establishment of the Society for the Treatment of Chronically Ill Children and the creation of children's clinics in Gatchina, Russia and Vindava, Latvia. During the revolutionary activity of 1905 in Russia, she agitated for the inclusion of women in whatever government might emerge from the political chaos.

Mariia Ivanovna Pokrovskaia (1852–*c.*1922)

Like Anna Shabanova, Mariia Pokrovskaia took advantage of the opening of the Women's Medical Courses in St Petersburg in 1873, joining in 1876 and graduating around 1882. She served for some time as a district physician in Pskov before returning to St Petersburg in 1888. She brought a statistical point of view to her analysis of living conditions among the poor, and in her writings, she connected issues of water, housing and air quality to the spread of urban diseases. She wrote a novel in 1903, *How I Was a City Doctor for the Poor*, that dramatised the hygiene problems facing the urban poor and made an appeal for more support for women medical practitioners. She was an organiser of the Women's Progressive Party during the revolutionary agitation of 1905, and edited and wrote for a feminist journal, *Women's Messenger*, which lasted until the revolutions of 1917.

Anna Ivanovna Veretennikova (1855–1888)

Yet another early graduate of the Women's Medical Courses in St. Petersburg, Veretennikova attended in 1877, a year after Pokrovskaia, and graduated in 1882. Like Pokrovskaia, she elected to spend her immediate post-college years serving as a district physician, but unlike Pokrovskaia, she chose a posting in the remote Ufimsk province, tending to non-Russian-speaking Muslims, occupying a one-room hut that served as her office as she attempted to stretch the meagre resources allotted her to a population hungry for medical treatment. Frustrated at the lack of official support, she returned to St Petersburg, where she worked in an eye clinic until her early death at the age of 33.

Bertha van Hoosen (1863–1952)

In 1915, Bertha van Hoosen and Marion Craig Potter founded the American Medical Women's Association to advocate for women's role in medicine and support women medical professionals. Van Hoosen served as the first president of the organisation. She had received her medical degree from the University of Michigan in 1888, but faced persistent discrimination in her subsequent career, which prompted her to create an organisation that would aid women who were struggling in isolation to navigate a career in medicine.

Flora Pollack (1865–1938)

Flora Pollack was a US physician known for her five-year study of venereal disease in children which uncovered the prevalence of men acting upon the 'infectionist theory' that held that syphilis could be cured by passing it on to a virgin, prompting those men to commit acts of sexual assault on minors. She also studied the effect of syphilis on rates of miscarriage and premature birth. As a result of her studies, a public information campaign was begun to educate the population about social hygiene and issues surrounding the transmission and nature of syphilis.

Chapter 19

A Doctor at Sky's Edge

Susan Anderson and the Practice of Medicine on America's Last Frontier

Seventy miles west of Denver, in a small town nestled 8,574 feet above sea level there rests the town of Fraser. Today an enclave of 1,400 hearty souls it was, in 1907, one of the United States' last wild places; the home of stout Scandinavian lumberjacks and the brave-unto-foolhardy men who operated the rickety, avalanche-prone train line over the Rocky Mountains. That year there arrived in Fraser an anomaly in more senses than one – a small tubercular woman doctor seeking to escape a run of bad fortune, all alone save for a small dog that followed her everywhere and snapped at everyone.

Her name was Dr Susan Anderson and her life to that point had not been a happy one. Her father, William Anderson, was by turns domineering and paternally attentive and, after he divorced his wife, Marya Pile, five years after Susan's birth in 1870, and took both Susan and her younger brother John with him to Wichita, Kansas, his was to be her sole parental influence. In Wichita, William was regarded as a fine veterinarian, and he cherished high ambitions that one of his children might become a doctor. Susan showed both higher intellectual promise than her somewhat diffuse brother, and greater drive, and when she declared in her teens an ambition to be a telegraph operator, William purchased a book for her, *What Women Can Do*, by way of encouraging her to set her goals higher.

John and Susan went to grammar school together, but when it came time for Susan to attend high school in Wichita proper, William declared that she must wait two years for her brother to catch up to her so that they could go to school together, and she dutifully complied, teaching at the grammar school she had just graduated from, and waiting for John. A stellar student at Wichita, she graduated in 1891 at the age of 21, just in time to have her life turned upside down by two momentous events.

The first of these was her father's marriage to a woman by the name of Minnie, only a few years the senior of Susan. In the years to come,

Minnie worked concertedly to divert as many resources as possible away from William's first two children and towards her own, almost derailing the completion of Susan's medical education in the process. That tendency, however, seemed a minor irritant at first next to William's sudden decision in 1892 to move to Cripple Creek, Colorado, where massive gold deposits had just been discovered. Among the first settlers of the area, William made the prudent decision to make his money not in mining for gold but in trading shares in prospective and already established mines.

William's business prospered while Susan experienced the discomfort of being one of a small handful of young women in a ramshackle town of rough prospectors. William disliked the marked attention they paid to his daughter almost as much as he disliked being caught in the middle of the regular fights between Susan and Minnie – two problems which could be solved at a stroke by sending Susan off to college at the University of Michigan-Ann Arbor. At the time, the student body was 25 per cent female, and all classes save anatomy were co-educational, a marked improvement over the situation several decades prior, when Elizabeth Blackwell and her successors began the fight for women's medical education. The cost to attend was a whopping $35 per semester (at the time an average semi-skilled worker could expect to make, depending on the region, about $1.25 a day), which was manageable so long as William's business prospered, but the year Susan entered Ann Arbor was also the year of the great Panic of 1893, and soon Minnie was remonstrating with William to cut off Susan and John's college funds.

William sent a letter to Susan, explaining that, as John had not been making full use of his expensive education in California, it was senseless to keep spending money for it, and that, if John was no longer getting an education, it was 'only fair' that she stop attending Ann Arbor as well and return home to Cripple Creek. She refused, and thanks to a wealthy friend, was able to continue paying for her last years at the college. She worked hard as a medical student on the night shift at Catherine Street Hospital, pushing herself through sleepless nights, and taking every opportunity to watch surgical methods.

During her last year at Ann Arbor, she contracted tuberculosis, with its accompanying fits of coughing and weakness and the grim likelihood of a much-truncated lifespan. Susan returned to Cripple Creek in 1897 to set up a small practice in a town already possessing too many medical practitioners, many of whom were little more than itinerant quacks. Her practice was small, but by 1900 life seemed to be on the up and up. A mysterious gentleman with the initials of W. R. had proposed marriage, and her loveable, if perpetually under-achieving, brother had moved back into town.

Then, dual tragedy struck. After a mysterious conversation with her father, W. R. suddenly pulled out of the proposed marriage, and in March John contracted pneumonia. William and Minnie did not inform Susan of his sickness right away, and by the time they did call her to treat him, there was nothing left to be done; on 16 March, John passed away, leaving Susan suddenly very alone in the world.

She left Cripple Creek, the site of so much loss and conflict, intent on making her own way as a doctor. She set up practice first in Denver, in 1901, but as a newly arrived woman doctor suffering from tuberculosis, she failed to make much headway and was ultimately compelled to accept a position as a nurse in Greeley, Colorado, where she was resented by the other nurses for her superior education. Her tuberculosis was not improving, and the crush of a 1907 diphtheria epidemic stretched her reserves of energy and mental fortitude to the breaking point.

The previous year, she had spent a blissful slice of time in the town of Fraser, where the air was so thin, cool and dry, that her fragile lungs could breathe it to their content. Perched high atop the world, peopled by colourful characters, set in an atmosphere of crisp mountain beauty, it seemed the ideal place to go to recover her strength and sanity after the buffeting she had received at Greeley.

She was noticed immediately after stepping off the platform at Fraser – an attractive if frail 37-year-old woman setting foot in a town dominated by Swedish lumberjacks, hired to clear the virgin forests, and poor miners working to blast a way through the mountainside to provide a safer alternative to the existing and ludicrously underserviced rail line. The local rumour mill soon established that she was in fact a doctor, and though she did not set out immediately to practise medicine, she was soon sought out by a man in wide-eyed panic, demanding that she must come to his house to save 'Dave', who had been caught up in barbed wire. She went with the man to his property, only to find that Dave was, in fact, a horse, and that seemingly the entire town had gathered to see what this small, tuberculosis-ridden woman could possibly do to cure him.

Annoyed at the deception, Susan saw a suffering creature before her and set to work, sterilising her equipment, issuing orders and setting herself the dangerous task of stitching together the multiple gashes across the legs and flank of a massive, frightened farm horse. One errant kick could have meant the end of Dr Susan Anderson at that point, but the locals noted with admiration how she stayed at her task until it was completed to her exacting standards. Word got out fast – Dr Anderson, or Doc Susie as she insisted on being addressed, knew her stuff.

For the next half a century, Susan Anderson gained for herself a reputation as the best rural doctor in the territory. She was so beloved by the Scandinavian lumberjack community that, when she was kicked out of the shack she lived in by the railroad company that owned the right of way through it, dozens of Swedes descended on a patch of territory that had been donated to her, and made a day of erecting a home and doctor's office thereupon to her exacting specifications, as a way of thanking her for all of the work she had done for them.

When she took patients over the mountains to the nearest city hospital, her opinion was treated with dignified respect by doctors there who earned more in a week than she did in a year. In fact, one of their favourite instructive pranks to play on interns unfamiliar with Doc Susie was to watch as they put on airs when she entered the hospital in her rough, practical country clothes with a patient in tow, and proceeded to dictate to her what her patient *really* ailed of, only to have Anderson's original diagnosis routinely proven correct upon closer examination. The doctors thought it an excellent lesson in humility and respect for their cocky young charges.

In 1926, Susan Anderson was sworn in as coroner for Grand County, a post which brought some much-needed extra money into her pockets while also placing her in the centre of the ongoing debate over worker safety at the construction site for the great Moffat Tunnel, a 6.2-mile-long project conceived by industrialist David Moffat, and seen through at breakneck speed by William Freeman, whose neglect for basic safety precautions along the existing line was legendary.

Anderson spoke up about the need to pay attention to the unpublished tragedies connected with the construction of the tunnel, that the casualties were not limited to those who perished in the occasional tunnel collapse, but included those wounded and poisoned in the long course of their work in ways that never made the papers. When the tunnel was first opened in 1928, and the wives of the tunnel and railroad workers were not given seats on the first train through in order to make room for the dignitaries chosen by the regional newspaper, the *Denver Post*, she placed herself at the tunnel's mouth with a collection of brave locals and workers, and wrote in large letters on a sign big enough for Freeman to see from his seat on the first car, 'WE BUILT THIS TUNNEL THE POST DIDN'T.'

Several times over the ensuing decades, Anderson considered moving to a more hospitable clime out East, and just as often she found herself unable to leave behind the town that had come to rely upon her rigorous efficiency and kind heart. She had brought the techniques of modern medicine, including thorough sterilisation procedures, to groups of men who had been treated as essentially expendable up to that point, and groups of women who expected little more than silent and monotonous suffering as their lot in life. She continued serving as a doctor in Fraser until 1956, finally retiring at the age of 86, and resided in that town until 1958, when her colleagues at Colorado General Hospital took over her end-of-life care, seeing to it that Colorado's most distinguished frontier doctor (Ethel Barrymore had inquired after the rights to making her life into a movie) came to an end as peaceful as her long and often arduous life most decidedly deserved. Dr Susan Anderson died on 16 April 1960, in a rest home in Denver, Colorado.

Further Reading

Virginia Cornell is the historian who did the work gathering the pieces of Dr Anderson's story together from letters, newspaper profiles and local Colorado records. Her book, *Doc Susie: The True Story of a Country Physician in the Colorado Rockies* (1991) is probably in the top ten of flat-out most enjoyable Women In Science reads you are likely to come across, full of big characters, forbidding landscapes, as well as personal, familial and professional drama of the most eternally compelling sort. Plus, it has perhaps my favourite end of a chapter yet written, concluding the chapter about the treatment of Dave the Horse:

> 'It was an era when house calls were common. But Doc Susie's first medical case in Fraser was a horse call.'

Chapter 20

Lymph, There it is

Florence Sabin, Pioneer Woman of Medical Research

For women in science, posterity has three fates in store. Some, like Marie Curie or Rosalyn Yalow, are recognised in their time and remain that way in the history books. Others, like Mary Anning or Marie Tharp, have to wait for later generations to rediscover them. And then there is that curious third category, of women hailed as geniuses in their lives who, for some reason, we have grown to forget. Florence Sabin (1871–1953) is, sadly, one such.

While living, she was showered with accolades, and books of her life and work appeared regularly in the ensuing decades. As it stands now, however, a major biography devoted to Sabin has not come out for forty long years. She broke through every barrier there was to assemble from nothing a career spanning three different areas of research, and for some reason, we have decided as a planet that we cannot be bothered with her any more. It is a case of really unfathomable neglect, and it is time we fixed it.

Florence Sabin was, plainly put, everything that is good and noble about science. She loved research, and was passionate about doing it correctly, but also recognised the world outside of the laboratory, devoting herself to issues of public health and education. She believed that a scientist needed to keep abreast of cultural and political developments, and made sure to arrange evenings for her students where they could listen to musicians and writers wrestling with the issues of the day.

As a person, she was admirable, and as a scientist, remarkable. She rewrote our knowledge of the lymphatic system, then shifted gears to discover unknown components of our immune response, before devoting herself to the chemistry of tuberculosis. And then, AND THEN, in her late seventies she accepted a political appointment to remake the entire state of Colorado's health system, directly saving tens of thousands of lives with her tireless lecture appearances and public health lobbying.

That phenomenal life began with all the drama and tragedy inherent in American frontier life. Her father was intending to go into medicine when word of a gold strike in Colorado distracted him. Moving Out West, he took up work as a mine manager and met a schoolteacher from his native Vermont who was likewise a recent Colorado immigrant. They married and had two daughters in quick succession, Mary and our Florence, and then the typical nineteenth-century Western cavalcade of horrendous tragedy rolled into town. Their next child died. Undeterred, they tried again and, after the next birth, Florence's mother died. The resulting child lived about a year, then died. Moving in with relatives, she met her grandparents, and grew to love them, *just* in time for the grandmother to die.

Her father, away from home too often to properly care for his two surviving daughters, sent them at first to a boarding school and then to live with their uncle, who noted Florence's gift for music and supported it. Until her junior year at the Vermont Academy, in fact, she was sure that her future was going to be that of a pianist. And then one day, as Florence was practising, some Mean Girl strode in and asked her to play something with a melody in place of her incessant piano exercises. Florence refused, saying she needed to practise technique if she was going to be a concert performer, to which Mean Girl replied that Florence was, at best, a gifted amateur, and could never make the professional cut.

It was an ungracious thing to say, but probably true, and Sabin knew it. After a dark night of soul-searching, she decided that she needed to devote her considerable energies to something else, and hit upon the idea of graduating college with honours, and concluded that science was the ideal place to apply her unique gifts of perseverance and curiosity. She shone in her classes and decided upon a career in medicine after hearing that Johns Hopkins University, on the occasion of a sizable donation from a group of proto-feminists, had been compelled to accept women as medical students on an equal basis with men.

Unfortunately, with her father's gold mines failing, Sabin could count on no parental financial support and so, for the next three arduous years, she scrimped and saved every penny she earned through tutoring and teaching to finally buy herself an education at Johns Hopkins. It was the right decision from the first. Her instructors noted her zeal, self-direction, and flawless laboratory technique. Like Rita Levi-Montalcini a generation later, she came to the notice of her professor, Dr Franklin Paine Mall, through the precision of her slide and staining preparations. Seeing the makings of a true research scientist in her, he gave her the task of creating a new model of the midbrain for instructional purposes. Her carefully wrought model was so precise, and contained so many features as yet unnoticed by neuroscience, that she was commissioned to change it into a book, *An Atlas of the Medulla and Midbrain*, which remained a standard text for years to come.

As important as the brain atlas was (and let's all just appreciate that her first project was Mapping. … THE BRAIN), it was Mall's next assignment that brought her to national prominence. For a long time, a controversy had raged in anatomical circles about how the lymphatic system developed, and what precisely it did. Mall set Sabin the task of meticulously studying lymphatic system formation in whatever manner she saw fit. The designing and implementing of the study were entirely her own, and for the next decade, she set about uprooting all of biology's most cherished notions about this mysterious entity. She decided to study smaller embryos than had been used before to give her a better view of the early stages of the lymphatic system's development, and, in a flash of insight, used Indian ink as the staining agent in place of the more traditional but coarser-grained Berlin blue. The combination worked and allowed her to see that, contrary to popular belief, the lymphatic system emerged from the blood vessels and spread into the intracellular space, rather than vice versa. The establishment would fight her fiercely for overthrowing their cherished doctrine, and would not hesitate to use the fact that she was a woman to try and have her data thrown out, but through careful experimentation and a refusal to be cowed, she won the day and established the basis of modern lymphatic theory.

With her work equally lauded and reviled, Sabin was already a figure of international scope, before even graduating, and was given the option to either carry out a one-year term at Johns Hopkins hospital, or to receive a special grant to carry on research under Dr Mills. She felt it would be a bigger step for the cause of women in science if she accepted the hospital residency, and discovered while there how very much she did not want to be a medical doctor. She hated the alternation between high pressure (births and surgeries) and mechanical repetition (paperwork and prescriptions), and decided to return to research for good. Upon finishing her year, Mall fought to get her an assistantship at Johns Hopkins which turned into an associate professorship. She was his second in command, an inspiring classroom lecturer and accessible mentor to all the students, and when Mall died, she should have succeeded to his position.

Instead, the spot went to a subordinate professor who had the jolly good sense to have been born male. Sabin was offered a less-prestigious full professorship in histology, but the snub rankled, and when she was offered a chance to transfer her new studies on white blood cells to the Elysian

Fields of the Rockefeller Institute, she grabbed the opportunity. Leaving teaching was not easy, but the chance to do fully funded research around the clock on the important problem of discovering the causes and cure for tuberculosis was irresistible. While there, she did foundation-laying work on the biochemistry of the disease, including the discovery of the fatty acid responsible for the development of tuberculosis's tell-tale tubercles and an extension of her previous studies of monocytes, a white blood cell she had discovered while at Johns Hopkins.

Her team did not *cure* tuberculosis, but they clarified the constituents of its major features, and elements of its growth and development, which paved the way for the later drug therapies that would finally take the disease off the list of perennial American killers. Her research was cut short, firstly by mandatory retirement at the age of 65, and secondly by the declining condition of her sister, Mary, which necessitated a move back to Colorado, and six mind-numbing years of retirement.

But it was not the end for Sabin! Some bright politicians in Colorado thought it would be a fine idea to appoint her to head a new department of health. After all, she was old and famous, and probably too feeble to cause much trouble. They reckoned wrong. Given purpose again, Sabin sprang into action, and uncovered the shocking state of Colorado public health. In deaths caused by the most prominent but preventable transmittable diseases of the day, it ranked consistently in the bottom five, and its record of regulating the dairy industry was nothing short of abysmal. Though nearing 80, Sabin travelled from town to town, giving people the shocking statistics and letting them know what they could do if they wanted pure milk and uncontaminated water again. The people of Colorado loved her, and every politician who backed her health programme was handily re-elected, helping her push through a series of reforms which vastly improved the quality of life in the state.

Meanwhile, her sister's health was failing, but Sabin did not have the heart to send her to a nursing home, and chose to take on the sleepless burden herself, the result being that she wrecked her own health, and Mary had to go to a nursing home anyway. Physically exhausted, Florence Sabin was checked into the hospital in 1953, there to die from a heart attack while watching her favourite team, the Brooklyn Dodgers, play the hated New York Yankees. She had penetrated the mysteries of anatomy, been friends with Gertrude Stein, given an entire state its health back, and won every accolade and degree there was to win in the medical profession, and yet the last thing she heard in this life was that her team was down by five points.

Further Reading

After Sabin's death, there were a number of good books produced trying to sum up her remarkable contributions to American medicine. *Florence Sabin: Colorado Woman of the Century* by Elinor Bluemel (1959) is perhaps the most famous, but my preferred source comes ten years later, with *Probing the Unknown: The Story of Dr Florence Sabin* by Mary Kay Phelan. If you have a pre-teen who is interested in scientists, it is a great book to thrust into their hands. More recently there have been some books routinely weighing in at fewer than 100 pages. *Florence Sabin: Medical Researcher* (1990) is a young adult title that does not back down from talking about monocytes and fibrous tissues, which is nice.

Chapter 21

'I Doubled My Fist' Sara Josephine Baker and the Fight for Child Hygiene

How deep can hopelessness go? Is there a lower limit, a solid floor against which we can push and thrust ourselves back into some semblance of striving humanity? Or does it just keep going down? Perhaps that hard line comes with the having of children – that no matter how much you have lost hope for yourself, nonetheless you will keep trying and struggling with whatever fight is left in you to keep those children alive and well.

Would it were so, but the bottomlessness of despair even amidst dizzying prosperity is something we only have to look back a century to behold in all of its fetid glory: to the early 1900s, and the tenements of New York. Six thousand souls crammed into a block of tin-shack housing with workers sleeping in shifts on piles of insect-ridden and rotting hay, dulling the pain with drink and oblivious to anything but the wear of the day, while sore-ridden pregnant and physically abused mothers lay in dank rooms waiting to give birth to children likely to die in a matter of weeks. Here hope was in slight supply. Infant mortality spiralled to levels unknown anywhere in the developed world while corrupt public health officials declared the problem unsolvable and therefore not worth wasting effort or resources upon.

It was into this world of calamitous infant death and official indifference that Dr Sara Josephine Baker (1873–1945) arrived like a meteor at the turn of the twentieth century. Efficient and incorruptible, she drummed out health workers who refused to sully themselves with tenement work and established the world's first Bureau of Child Hygiene and along the way erected a string of institutions that formed the basis of modern infant care. All told, her efforts are estimated to have saved at least 90,000 babies directly, and her programmes became the model for child hygiene the world over.

For all the direct confrontation with death and disease that would form the heartbeat of her adult life, Baker's early years were the idyllic stuff of a Norman Rockwell painting. Born in Poughkeepsie, New York in 1873 in a well-off but not grotesquely wealthy family of Quaker stock to a lawyer father and a mother who was one of the first attendees of Vassar College, she enjoyed access to the example of educated women and the social calendar of Gilded Age youth. She alternated trips to New York City with rollicking country vacations featuring clam bakes, toboggan rides and drives in the back of hay wagons while singing 'Tea for Two' with groups of chums.

She even boasted a great aunt, a secret radical Quaker, who gathered the children about her while their parents were away to read them Bible stories in a dramatic voice only, at the end, to close the book with a thump and declare:

> Now children, that is a very silly story. I am an old, old lady and I want all of you to remember what I am saying. It is a silly story and there is not a word of truth in it. Do not ever let anyone tell you that stories like that are true … Jane! Cookies!

At which point cookies duly appeared and the children revelled in the sugar and the exposure to a grand old woman instilling in them the courage to think for themselves in spite of the Generally Accepted Truths.

Had life continued in that vein, Baker would have gone to Vassar, and comfort, and distinction of a certain sort, but fate dealt its long-delayed ultimate blow in her sixteenth year as she lost in quick succession her only brother and then her father. In an instant, the family went from sure economic comfort to a clawing panic as the household of women worried over what was to be done. Baker's sister was a virtual invalid, so Sara took it upon herself to find a job that would support the family. Giving up her dreams of Vassar, she scooped up what remained of the family's money and put it towards a seemingly mad plan to become a medical doctor by studying at the New York Infirmary Medical College.

All her acquaintances and relatives advised against the plan, but that only stiffened her stubborn resolve to see it through. Living in cheap rooms and eating as inexpensively as possible, she applied herself to the task of learning medicine at the establishment that had been founded a short three decades before by none other than Elizabeth and Emily Blackwell to provide medical training for women. It was a hard road, with ultimate financial success anything but certain, but after graduating in 1898, Baker found her niche relatively quickly, her practice growing as much by virtue of a youthful optimism that does not know what Can and Cannot Be Done as her own enterprising spirit.

While building up her private practice, in 1901 Baker entered the profession that would become her life's work when she accepted a job as a Department of Health medical inspector and came face to face with the insufficiency of the government's child health monitoring. School inspection programmes were farcical in their lack of thoroughness, and when illness was discovered, there were no resources to follow through on the cases. School nurses did not exist. Tenement inspectors routinely dodged their duties by making up rosy data about slum children in order to avoid having to do anything about it. Infant blindness ran rampant. Milk was not routinely pasteurised, and mothers would ladle it directly from store vats that crawled with bacteria only to then serve it from rusted cans. In the summer months, 1,500 babies died *weekly* from dysentery related diarrhoeal dehydration.

Baker resolved to do her job as it was meant to be done, in spite of the protests from her fellow inspectors that her conscientious thoroughness was ruining their system. She went into every building and viewed with horror the indifference to life all around her, the mothers so used to the deaths of their children that they could not be roused to efforts in caring for the next one in line. One episode from her autobiography speaks to the general tenor of her experience as an inspector:

> I thought I already knew something about how filthy a tenement room could be. But this was something special, particularly in the amount of insect life. One dingy oil lamp, by the light of which I could barely make out the woman in labor, lying on a heap of straw in the corner. Four stunted children, too frightened to make any noise, huddled together in a far corner. The floor was littered with scraps of food, too old to be easily identifiable, but all contributing to the odor of the place. Cockroaches and bedbugs crawled about everywhere. The only thing to wash up in was, as usual, an old tin basin, rusted and ragged at the edge. All of it was the nth power of abject, discouraged squalor. But the ugliest detail was a man, also lying on the floor because he was apparently too drunk to get up. But he was all too capable of speech.
>
> The moment I approached my patient I discovered that her back was one raw, festering sore. She said that her husband had thrown a kettle of scalding water over her a few days before. That accusation brought him to his feet crazy with rage, threatening me and her, toppling and lurching all over the place.
>
> I knew that could not go on. I had to get him out of the way. As he wavered toward me, waving his clenched fist and

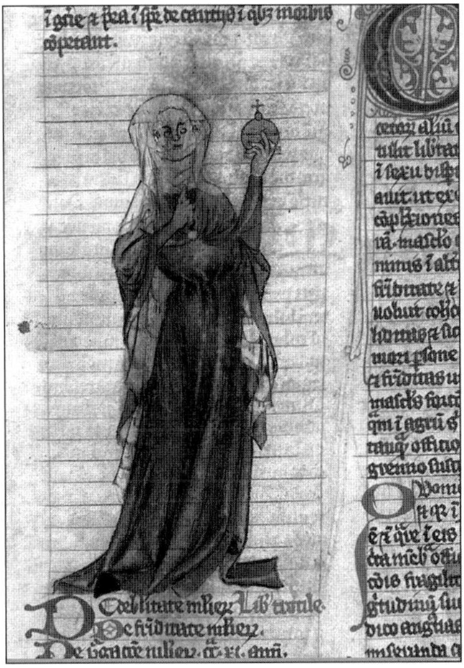

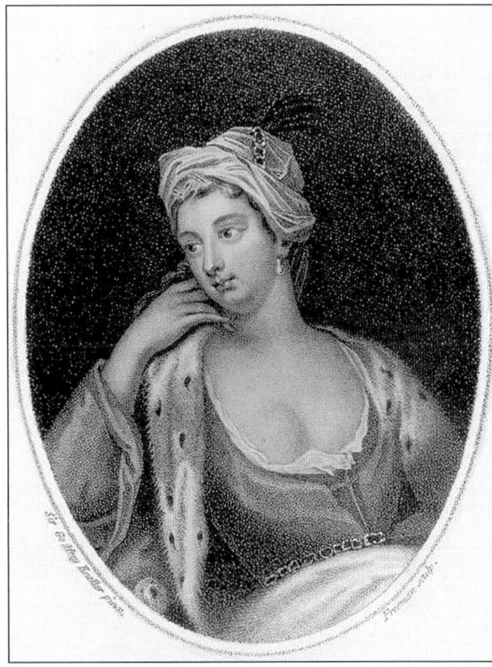

Above left: Trota of Salerno broke from Galenic theory to advocate for practical solutions to women's health issues gathered from multiple medical traditions. (Wikimedia Commons)

Above right: Lady Mary Montagu brought the technique of inoculation from the Ottoman Empire to England in the Eighteenth Century. (Wikimedia Commons)

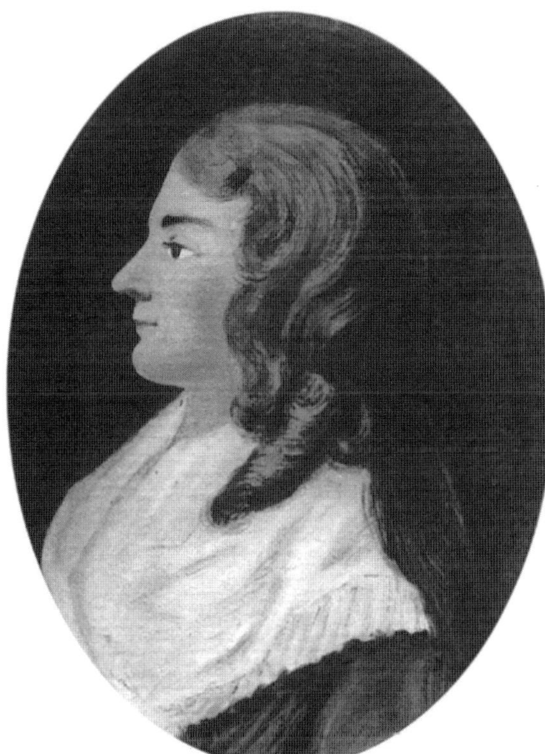

Right: Dorothea Erxleben received her medical degree in 1754, but it would be another century and a half before Germany began awarding such degrees to women again. (Wikimedia Commons)

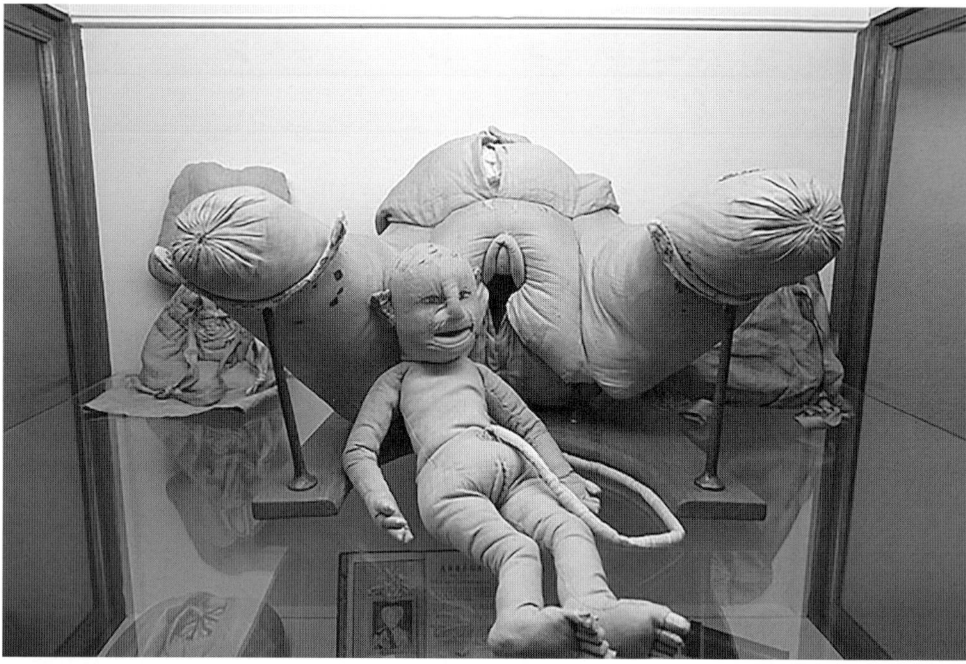

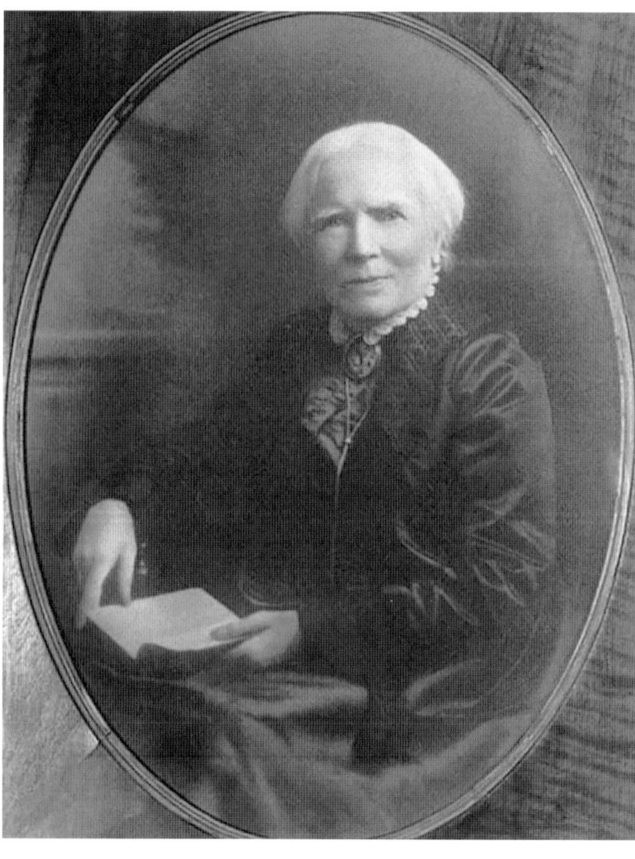

Above: One of Madame du Coudray's original birth demonstration models for teaching rural midwives how to approach different infant malpresentations. (Wikimedia Commons)

Left: The first English woman to obtain a medical degree, by this point in life Elizabeth Blackwell was largely isolated from the movement she had created. (Wikimedia Commons)

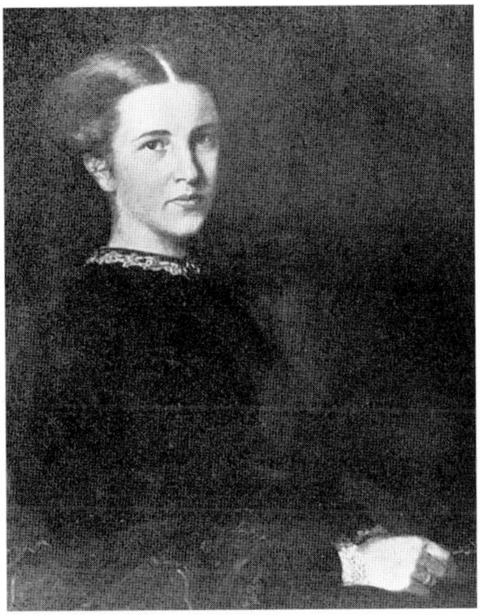

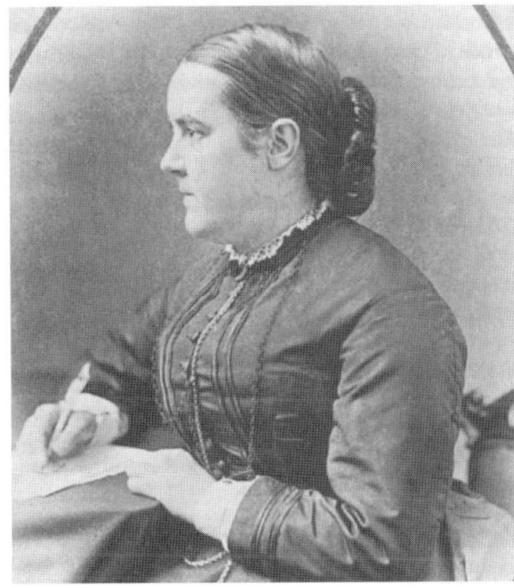

Above left: The leader of the Edinburgh Seven, Jex-Blake used every legal and rhetorical means at her disposal to further the cause of women's medical education. (Wikimedia Commons)

Above right: Elizabeth Garrett Anderson was Jex-Blake's polar opposite in approach to women's education, advocating for a gradualist, rather than confrontational, strategy. (Wikimedia Commons)

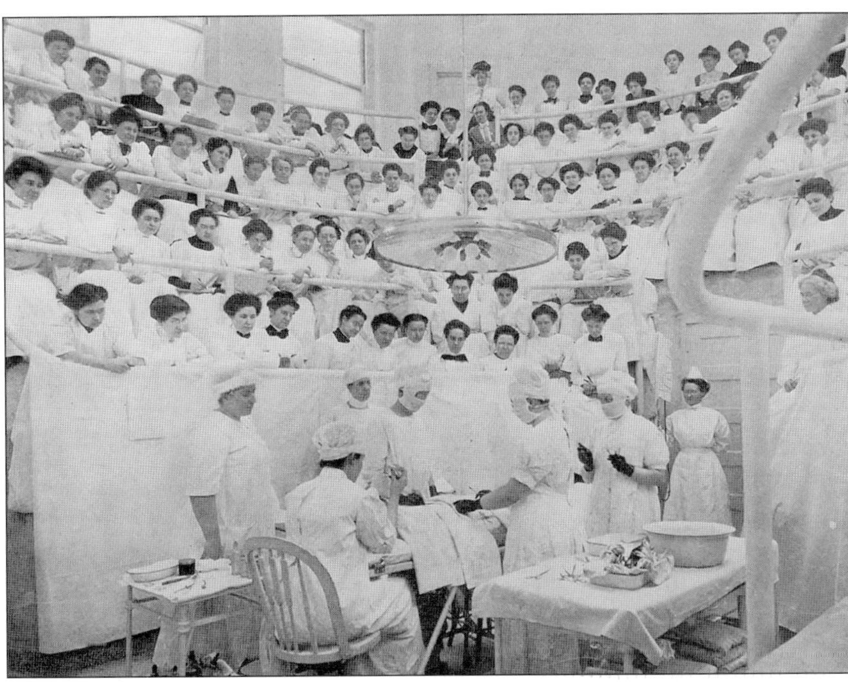

The newly constructed medical amphitheater at the Woman's Medical College of Pennsylvania, *c*. 1911. (Wikimedia Commons)

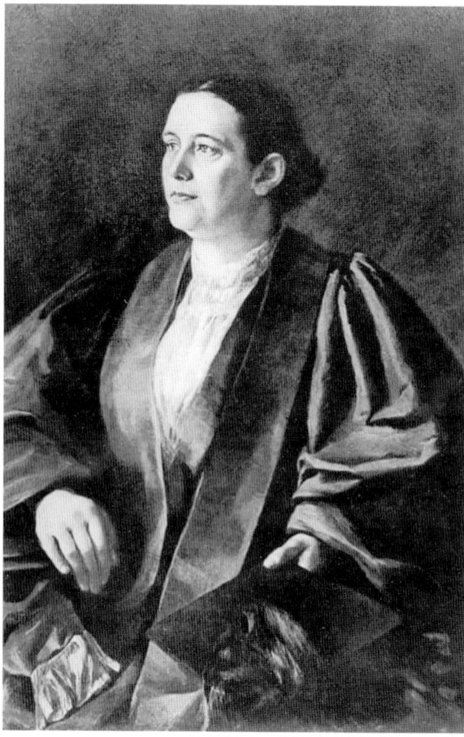

Edith Pechey-Phipson was a key figure in the fight to bring women's medical education to India in the late nineteenth century. (Wikimedia Commons)

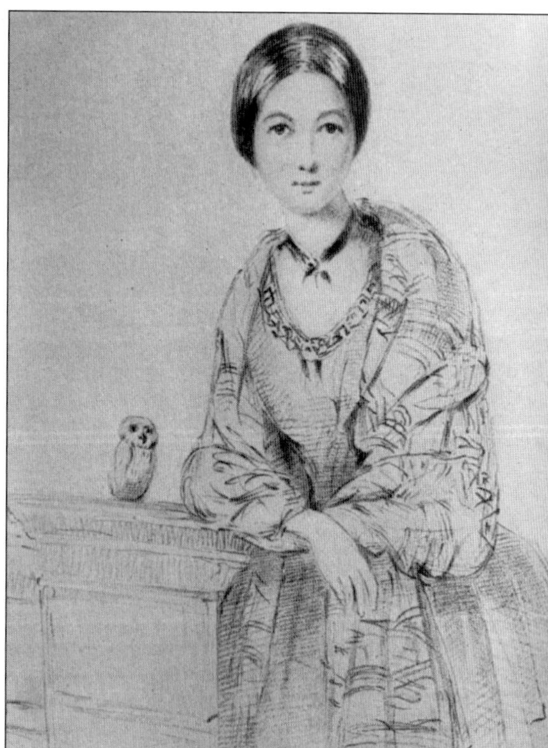

A drawing of Florence Nightingale after a portrait by Parthenope Lady Verney, featuring Nightingale with her tame owl, Athena. (Published in Cecil Woodham-Smith's 1951 biography of Nightingale)

Anandibai Joshee was the first Indian woman to receive a medical degree, though she died within a year of receiving it. (Wikimedia Commons)

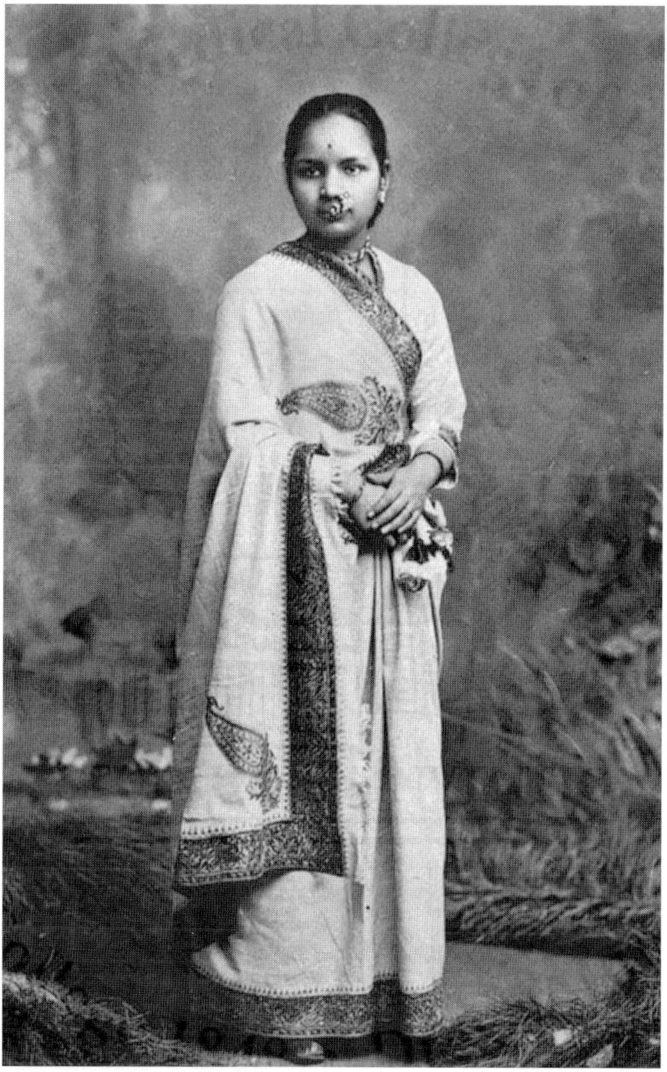

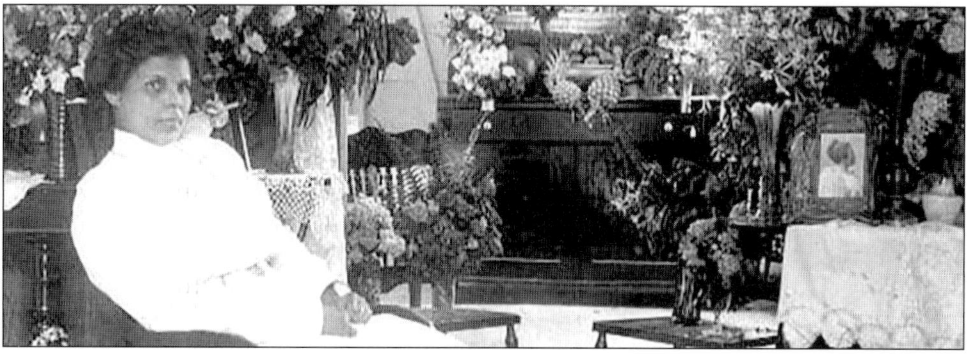

Picture of Dr Sarah Loguen Fraser at home in Puerto Plata, Dominican Republic, *c.* 1885. (Wikimedia Commons)

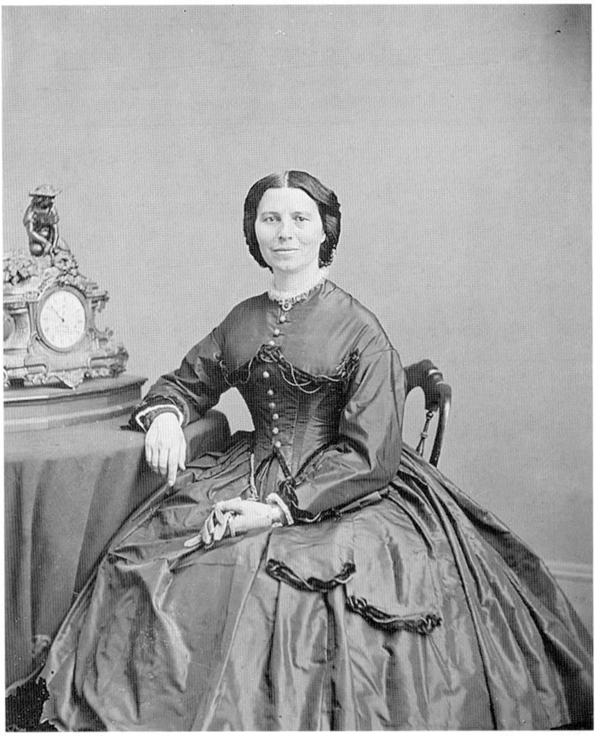

After her work during the United States Civil War, the 'Angel of the Battlefield' Clara Barton became the founder of the American Red Cross. (Wikimedia Commons)

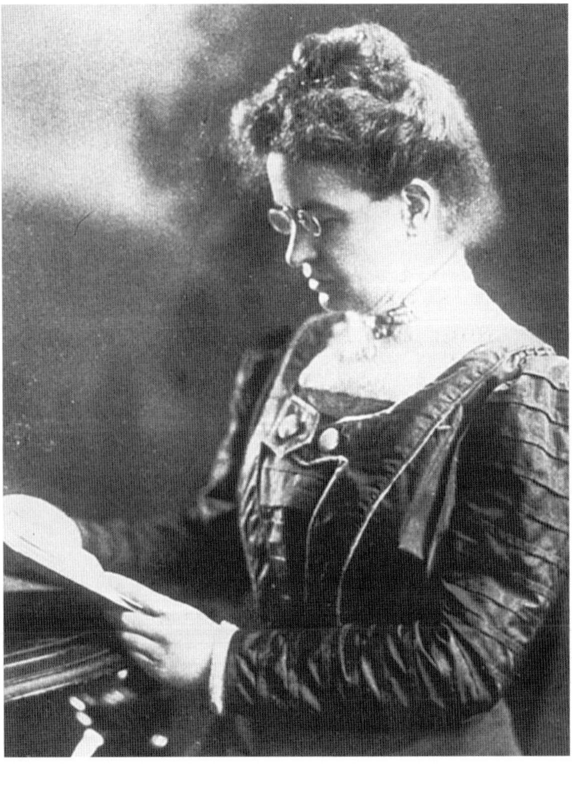

Medical researcher Florence Sabin made contributions to the study of the lymphatic system, and studied the biochemistry of tuberculosis. (Wikimedia Commons)

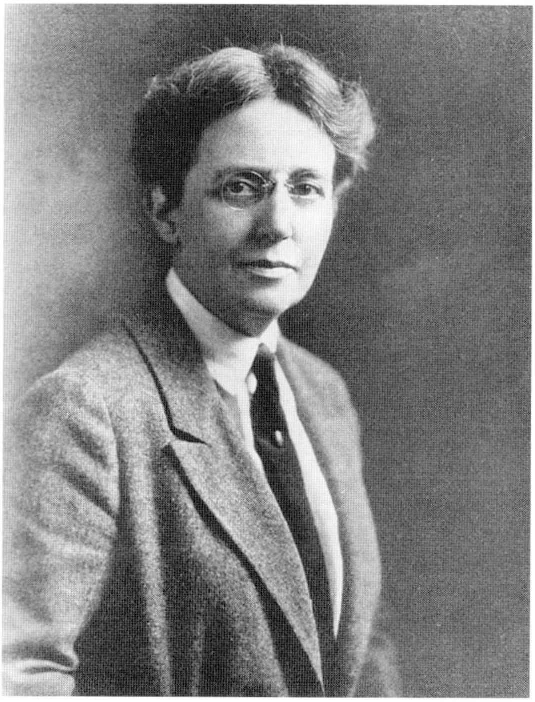

Sara Josephine Baker was a tireless advocate for better public health policies in the teeming tenements of early twentieth-century New York. (Wikimedia Commons)

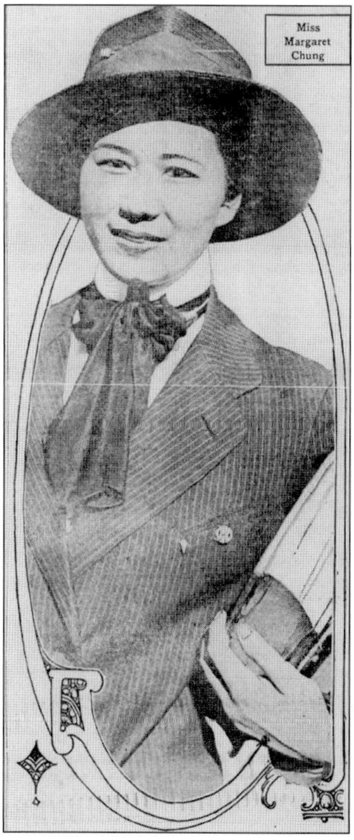

Margaret Chung was the first American-born Chinese woman to receive a medical degree, and went on to become a national celebrity during the Second World War. (Wikimedia Commons)

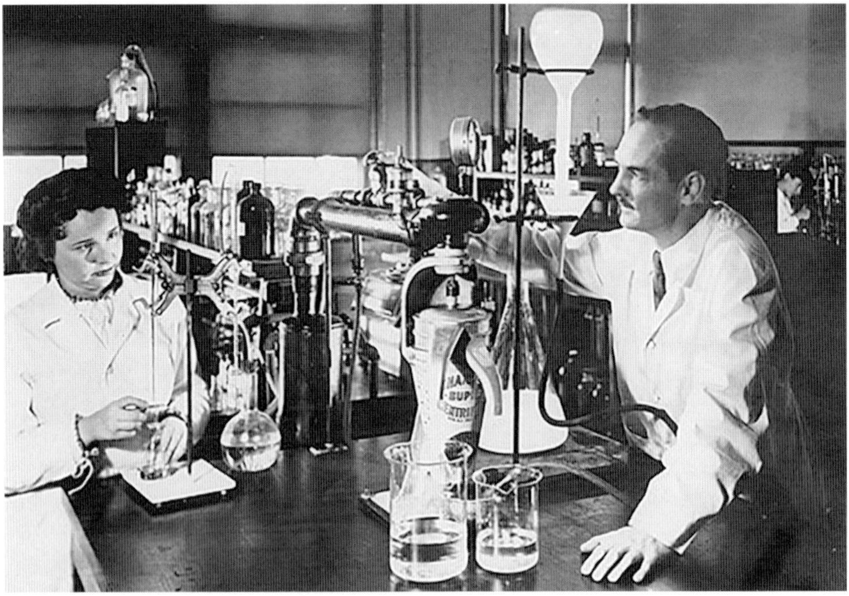

Gertrude Elion won the Nobel Prize for her development, with George Hitchings, of new medicine creation techniques centered on biochemical pathways. (Wikimedia Commons)

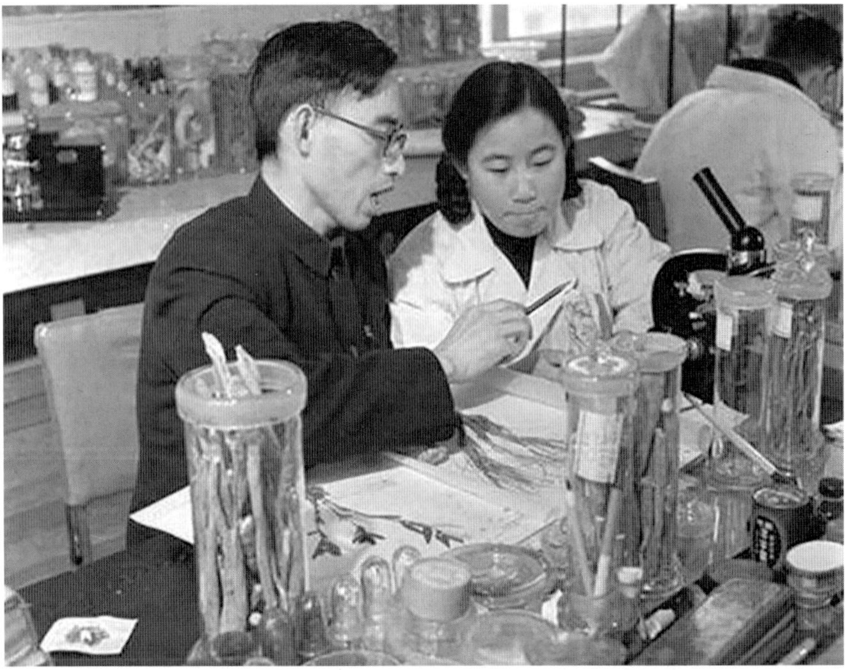

Tu Youyou, here shown some time in the 1950s, won the Nobel Prize for her development of the anti-malarial drug artemisinin, which has saved uncountable lives. (Wikimedia Commons)

> uttering verbal filth, I ran out into the hall. He followed as I had intended. I had thought of running in quickly again and seeing if the door would lock. But then, as he lurched after me, he crossed the stair-head and, with instinctive reaction, I doubled my fist and hit him. It was beautifully timed. I weighed hardly half as much as he, but he was practically incapable of standing up, and this frantic tap of mine was strategically placed. He toppled backward, struck about a third of the way down the rather long stair and slid to the bottom with a hideous crash.

The man survived, but was knocked out long enough to allow Baker to continue the delivery in peace. And that was but one episode on one day. Baker's reputation for honestly assessing and reporting the state of the tenements, while infuriating to her co-workers, caught the eye of her superiors, and she was slowly promoted to positions of higher authority until she had at last the power to act in substantial ways to improve the lives of infants and children, culminating in her role as director of the newly created Bureau of Child Hygiene from 1908 to her retirement in 1923.

Her accomplishments during these years represent a cavalcade of good sense pushed vigorously forward in the face of governmental confusion and medical resistance. Her insight was fundamental: if we devote resources to educating mothers about practices that prevent childhood diseases, we will not always be caught trying and failing to cure those diseases at their critical end stages. She argued with the city to fund projects in what we would now call preventive care, only to be derided by officials guffawing at the idea of spending money to cure people who were not sick.

She pushed on regardless, securing money from private industry when government would not come through, and working the strings of the Democratic party-political machine at Tammany Hall like a virtuoso when the situation called for it. She established a corps of visiting nurses to educate new mothers about hygienic practices, especially about access to fresh air and cool clothing in the summer months. Result: a decline in summer infant deaths by 1,200.

She wrangled some funding from private industry to create milk stations where mothers could get Grade A pasteurised milk at lower prices than they could buy Grade B from the stores, and while they were there, she made sure the staff taught them about the nutritional differences between cow's milk and breast milk, and how to supplement a child's diet if you did not breast feed. Result: the programme proved so successful and popular that the government was shamed into not only funding the existing stations but creating new ones as well.

She created a licensing system for midwives that gradually increased the training standards of that profession and allowed her to introduce the use of silver nitrate into midwife birth procedures which cut the instance of infant blindness from 300 cases yearly to three.

She took on the phenomenon of Little Mothers with sense and compassion. At the time, mothers who were breaking their backs to make ends meet often relied upon their eldest daughters to take care of the younger children in the family, with often tragic results. Baker started school programmes that met on Saturdays where these girls could learn more about how to take care of children properly, and how to address their own natural frustrations when things went wrong. The children learned, and were proud to pass their knowledge on to their parents and anybody else who would listen.

She *also* encouraged the first experiments with keeping nurses on staff at schools who were trained to deal with emergency situations and recognise illnesses that required the attention of specialists. She put a stop to a health board programme that invaded schools, lined the children up against the wall, sliced out their tonsils without anaesthetic or explanation, and then released them with blood flowing from their mouths, and replaced it with a series of centres that informed the child about the procedure, used anaesthetic and made her comfortable for a day afterwards in a nice bed with plenty of ice cream. In the face of the great influenza epidemic of the war years, she argued that keeping the children in schools was the best way to keep them from infection, and as a result, not only was New York the only city with open schools at the time but dramatically fewer children died of influenza.

Her success in the fields of preventive medicine, child nutrition, and disease recognition and treatment were so great that she brought the medical establishment on her head on a number of occasions, including this encounter which is so fantastically absurd in its bare admission of venality that it is worth a full reading:

> I have already described two or three occasions when my colleagues insisted on getting in our way for what seemed to us the worst of all possible bad reasons. But I never saw the short-sighted psychology of a certain type of doctor, when confronted with public health work, better brought out than by a representative of a New England medical society testifying

> before a Congressional committee which was considering the appropriation of funds for the newly founded Federal Children's Bureau. I was down there testifying too – on the other side. This New England doctor actually got up and told the committee: 'We oppose this bill because, if you are going to save the lives of all these women and children at public expense, what inducement will there be for young men to study medicine?' Senator Sheppard, the chairman, stiffened and leaned forward: 'Perhaps I didn't understand you correctly,' he said; 'You surely don't mean that you want women and children to die unnecessarily or live in constant danger of sickness so there will be something for young doctors to do?' 'Why not?' said the New England doctor, who did at least have the courage to admit the issue; 'That's the will of God, isn't it?'

These are but some of the institutions created from nothing by the insight and willpower of Sara Josephine Baker, and some of the prejudices she faced, both as a woman (her entire doctoral staff came to her when she was nominated director of the Bureau and threatened to resign en masse in protest for having to take orders from a woman until she talked them down) and as a worker for infant health in the face of large medical and governmental interests. And that is but a part of her story – she was also the person who tracked down renowned disease vector Typhoid Mary on two separate occasions; a suffragist who addressed sceptical crowds on street corners; an international observer who shamed America with an account of the superior scale of Soviet efforts to ensure the health of children; and a fashion icon whose uniform of a man's suit topped with a four-in-hand tie and a pair of TR pince-nez earned her the nickname of Dr Joe. A keen devotee of Theodore Roosevelt's advocacy of The Strenuous Life, she filled her time with work and public service, and her efforts attracted observers from every corner of the globe to see how much could be accomplished by a society dedicated to the proposition that infant life is of fundamental value.

She retired in 1923 from her directorship of the bureau and settled on a New Jersey farm in the 1930s with her partner, the Australian novelist Ida Wylie. Here she wrote her autobiography, *Fighting for Life*, in 1939, and a string of popular articles on health and child care besides. She died of cancer in 1945, having lived to see the experimental shoestring programmes of her youth and middle years become the standard practices of a nation, and a world.

Further Reading

Fighting for Life (1939) is that rare bird – a scientific autobiography of almost irresistible literary charm and dash. It is among the greatest science memoirs of all time. Its depiction of Gilded Age New York sizzles with electricity, just as her portrayals of tenement living are tone poems of dehumanisation. It is a book to read and then reread every decade or so to remind yourself of what we once were and how far we have come.

Chapter 22

Breaking the Shackles Procreative

Margaret Sanger and the Creation of the Pill

In 1912, it was against the law in the United States to publish a book that contained descriptions of birth control methods. It was against the law to even expound the theoretical benefits of birth control as a general notion. It was against the law to put a contraceptive diaphragm into the hands of a desperate mother of twelve in an attempt to save her life from serial pregnancy. It was against the law to give a woman a pamphlet that described how her own reproductive organs worked. And while the majority of reform-minded women of the era turned to the suffrage movement as their primary outlet of activity, one looked at the sea of poor mothers, drowning in unwanted pregnancy, bodies broken but without recourse, and decided to make the relieving of their suffering her life's work. Margaret Sanger (1879–1966), more than any other single individual in human history, is responsible for placing mankind's reproductive destiny back in the hands of those who bear its burdens.

She knew of what she spoke. She was born into a poor gravestone engraver's family to a mother who had been pregnant eighteen times in thirty years of marriage, seven of them miscarriages. And her family was in no way unique in Corning, a town that sustained itself on serving the local glassworks factory, the rambling immigrant houses teeming with children sent off to work at age 9 to earn just enough to not starve. Maggie Higgins was born in 1879, six years after the passage of a set of laws that had as their express purpose the perpetuation of this system of hopeless overpopulation.

In 1873, Anthony Comstock, self-appointed leader of the New York Society for the Suppression of Vice, made it his sanctimonious business to stamp out obscenity in the United States, and to that end crafted a series of laws, approved by Congress, to make it a crime to mail objectionable literature, or to distribute it. By his definition, anything that so much as mentioned birth control was an obscene affront to nature. Through his unflagging efforts, the Post Office was turned into a massive machine of censorship, refusing to deliver any periodicals that even abstractly hypothesised about the societal benefits of birth control, and anybody who distributed pamphlets privately on the topic was bound for as much as five years in jail. Women were to be kept fully ignorant of their own biologies, and entirely powerless to control their reproductive destiny. Thanks to the Comstock Laws, it was now legal in some states for a doctor to carry out an abortion, but illegal for him to distribute an informational pamphlet that might have avoided the pregnancy in the first place.

Higgins saw the results first hand as she trained to become a nurse in the late nineteenth century, treating the women wasting away from repeated unwanted pregnancy, and their malnourished children. Herself the daughter of an agnostic socialist, Higgins was disgusted with the role that religion played in perpetuating this misery for its own gains, and her radical tendencies only increased with her marriage to socialist sympathiser William Sanger in 1902. The marriage forced her to end her nurse's training, and the accusation of being an under-educated amateur in the health field would stalk her the rest of her days. Living in the heady world of New York socialist circles during America's last great flirtation with a worker-centred alternative to the two-party system, her association with radical authors, artists and devil-may-care libertines opened her eyes to a new mode of living.

She agitated for workers' causes, focusing at first on the economic woes of the industrial classes before coming to the realisation that many of the miseries of the modern-day world were ascribable to humanity's lack of control over its own fecundity. Wars, famine, urban crowding and capitalist exploitation all had their roots in our inability to voluntarily limit the number of offspring we produce. And religions, hungry for new followers, and companies, eager for cheap labour, and nations, desperate for cannon fodder, had all made it their concerted business to label the merest whisper of giving women control of their bodies as obscene and grotesque. In 1912, Sanger began her writing career in earnest with a series of articles, *What Every Girl Should Know,* for a socialist periodical. It advertised the desirability of promoting in a general way the cause of voluntary reproduction, without mentioning specifics as to methods, and even this vague mentioning of birth control was deemed too radical in the eyes of a government run mad on Comstockery.

One of the astounding things about Sanger, however, was her sheer resilience. No matter how many copies of her magazines were confiscated, how many of her clinics shut down, how many of her talks cancelled by weary Catholic-nudged local officials, and how many times she was dragged to stand trial for offering reproductive counsel to distraught married women, she only used the adversity to further what she believed was humanity's greatest cause. Often times utterly alone, forced to fill out her *Birth Control Review* with self-penned articles written under various pseudonyms, the object of derision not only of the conservative establishment but of other feminists who viewed her tactics as too radical and non-conciliatory, she gave every moment and every resource to organising and reorganising her movement, becoming a figure of only passing familiarity to her own children in the process.

For three long decades of slogging, all of her efforts amounted to a tragic pittance in the face of the titan she had sworn to combat. The Catholic Church used every weapon at its disposal to thwart any progress she managed by pure personal resolution to tear from the inertia of American prudery. Its close links with the police force allowed the Church to shut down her meetings and infiltrate her clinics with undercover police spies. Its lobbying might compelled presidents to turn against their own inclinations to embrace birth control in order to appease this important voting bloc. Everywhere she appeared, priests railed from pulpits against her affronting of God's plan, vehemently choosing airy doctrinal purity over actual human suffering.

Meanwhile, the medical community would officially have nothing to do with her or her cause. When she finally won the right to open advisory clinics if they were staffed by doctors rather than nurses and volunteers, she struggled to find somebody willing to ruin their career by associating with birth control. And as to her pet cause, the one for which she is most known, of developing an oral contraceptive, the medical establishment could not be bothered. The money was in thwarting infertility, not inducing it. So, it was up to Sanger, and her financial benefactor Katharine McCormick, to find scientists doing promising research and personally support their efforts against the indifference of the larger research community. Sanger's research into the problem revealed to her that the most likely approach would be a hormonal one, and that the most promising work was being done by Dr Gregory Pincus and Dr John Rock, the former of whom was teetering on the closure of his laboratory before McCormick and Sanger descended to rescue his work.

Pouring money and support into his research on progesterone as an interrupter of the ovulation cycle, and benefiting from the much laxer drug-testing policies of the era, Sanger was able to unveil the world's first birth control pill, Enovid, in 1957. Within two years, a million women would be using the product, and within a decade, the Supreme Court would strike down at last the Comstock Law that made birth control still illegal in states like heavily Catholic Massachusetts and Connecticut. Having spent four decades educating a reluctant and often ungrateful public as to their own biological interests, she lived to see a birth control revolution developed under her auspices achieve profound, if not general, acclaim.

In the history of birth control, Sanger is often considered as much an embarrassment as a leader. Her flair for publicity and organisation, the uncompromising way she approached the power of Church and nation, and her need for absolute control all set on edge the rank and file who wanted to professionalise the birth control movement, to make it something less aggressive and more media friendly. Sanger saw her Birth Control Clinical Research Bureau folded in with the American Birth Control League (one of the umpteen organisations she had previously created and left) to form Planned Parenthood, a name she abhorred as reeking of rosy committee-born wrong-headedness. Many of her cherished beliefs became hindrances to the later movement, including her early advocacy of eugenics, a set of ideas embraced by many Americans at the turn of the century. Whether she embraced it out of pure belief or out of a tactical need for allies in the struggling early days of birth control advocacy is an open question, but it remains a sore spot nevertheless, and the sense of 'Sanger? We'd rather not talk about *her*' is still palpable among those branches of reproductive history that would prefer a less idiosyncratic past.

But without Sanger, and the countless symposia she organised, the tens of thousands of people she helped face to face at her clinics, the reams of pages she wrote tirelessly expounding the principle of female reproductive self-determination, and her commitment to an inexpensive alternative to the irritating, cumbersome and ineffective diaphragms that had changed little since the days of the Egyptians, where would we be? She carried the torch when nobody else was willing, kept its basic principles alive through the unpromising days of war, and the heedless callousness of the Cold War's incessant post-bellum breeding. The pill would have come eventually without her concentrated guidance, but perhaps decades later, exposing another generation to the serial misery of wizened Victorianism wed to blind Catholicism. We can be who we are thanks to Margaret Sanger, who died in a retirement home, senile and in constant pain, just half a century ago.

Further Reading

Sanger wrote a couple of autobiographies, both of which had an eye towards propaganda and which routinely altered events (erasing the Jewish ancestry of her husband; completely ignoring her strings of lovers) to make the movement more credible. A better first book is undoubtedly Jean H. Baker's marvellous *Margaret Sanger: A Life of Passion* (2011). Sanger's quirky self-mythology is investigated rigorously but sympathetically, keeping in mind the demands of sustaining a movement nobody believed in against incredible odds over an entire lifetime. Sanger comes out an inspiring if complicated heroine, one who paid a heavy price, and enacted a heavy toll on those around her, for her eventual success.

Chapter 23

Milk and Blood

Icie Macy Hoobler and the Science of Infant-Mother Nutrition

A young mother of the early twentieth century who could not or did not want to breast feed was a creature entirely at the hands of bumbling chance. Doctors of the era prescribed individually concocted replacement formula recipes based on a mixture of patchwork research, folk wisdom and personal idiosyncrasy. The most scientific among them considered three factors and three alone: proteins, fats, and carbohydrates. The vitamin and antibody content of milk went blithely unmeasured until poor growth rates, scurvy and rickets became so endemic in lower-income households that a new, rigorous approach to infant nutrition, and the mother-foetus dyad, was required. The woman at the head of that approach was a pioneer farm-girl-turned-biochemist by the name of Icie Macy (1892–1984).

Her early life reads like a Laura Ingalls Wilder book. Born on a remote farm in Gallatin, Missouri in 1892, her first years were filled with the daily chores of rural life, with preparing food for preservation in the root cellar, harnessing horses for harvest, and occasionally mourning the passing of a beloved cow struck by lightning. Dirt roads, outhouses and country piety were the matter of her early memories – those, and a profound curiosity about nature's workings. *How* do seeds grow? *How* does a chick develop and hatch?

For many country girls, that curiosity went spectacularly unfulfilled, but Macy's parents believed stoutly in education and progress. Her father was at the head of every effort to bring technology to Gallatin, laying down electrical lines and paving roads, and he insisted that, so long as his daughter had the drive to learn, he would do whatever he could to ensure her the means. 'In the future we may not be able to provide you with many material things or wealth,' her parents said, 'but if we can encourage and provide an endowed education, we are giving you something that cannot be taken from you.'

Like Florence Sabin, her first dream was a musical career but, again like Sabin, she came to a point where she felt mere technical prowess could take her no further. She hated performing, and doubted her ability to meaningfully interpret the music beyond the correctness of the notes, and with her father's blessing switched her major from music to English. English, however, was a choice of convenience, as she came to realise her true passion lay in science, and in particular in the rapidly developing field of biochemistry. Her college career coincided with the heady days of the Vitamin Revolution, when the connection between vitamin deficiency and physical abnormality was being uncovered by a dedicated but often mocked cadre of scientists attempting to bring the insights of chemistry to the study of biology.

Macy was encouraged by her professors to not settle for a career as an under-appreciated teacher but to explore her gift for original research, and her early experiences in the classroom reinforced that decision. Though she attempted to make light of it, the daily harassment she endured as a woman science professor burns through the pages of her memoirs:

> In those years of my youth I blushed readily and radiantly. My associates and students had great fun in stimulating my red face and neck. At times I was forced to fight back to retain my womanly dignity and self-respect but usually I could muster some humor and accept the trauma without too much annoyance. Most of the students assigned to my sections of freshman chemistry were older than the usual freshman. Many were returning soldiers of World War I. Some resented having a woman teacher much less a young blushing upstart of a girl. Other students were less earnest and younger, were delighted to sit in the front row of seats looking up into the blushing face of their teacher, making wisecracks to increase the intensity of the color. This was traumatic at times until I regained my self-respect and gathered courage and determination to demonstrate to the class that a woman chemistry teacher was capable of teaching, even grown men just back from war.

Even when she was free of disrespectful students, her battle with casual institutional sexism was hardly done. As a researcher at a Pittsburgh hospital in 1920, she faced both of the undersung horrors of pioneering professional women: bathrooms and cafeterias.

It might sound trivial, but the roll call of absurd indignities experienced by early women scientists at the hands of these two facilities could fill its own chapter. Macy's case is a typical one. Her hospital had bathroom facilities for male staff only, and so informed her that, if she needed a restroom, she would have to use a public toilet a half-block away. That would involve leaving her post for an extended time and, since she did not want to get criticised for being absent, she did what so many women did in similar circumstances – she held it and only went to the toilet when absolutely necessary, developing an acute case of nephritis as a result that required months to recover from.

Meanwhile, in the cafeteria she was forbidden from eating with the male doctors, and regulations prevented her from eating with the nurses. So, a place was eventually found for her at the workers' cafeteria, except that her schedule did not match theirs, so she was reduced to eating whatever leftovers were to be had after their lunch, alone in an empty room.

She was, at this time, a doctor with a PhD from Yale, a highly gifted laboratory researcher doing important work in the emerging field of nutrition, and yet she was reduced to scavenging for leftovers, and ruining her kidneys, all for the sake of institutional prudery. It was a low point in her career and, though the president of the hospital eventually intervened on her behalf to remove the worst of the impositions, better times did not truly come until an offer arrived from UC Berkeley to teach under the expert guidance of home economics giant Agnes Fay Morgan.

She was not long in that post, however, before a call came from the newly established Merrill-Palmer School in Michigan to head their nutritional research division. That institution was established with the goal of improving the lot of children through a thorough study of the nutritional needs of mothers, foetuses and infants. It was an ideal job for Macy, with her focus on the intersection of children's welfare, chemistry and public policy.

Here, and at its successor institution, the Children's Fund of Michigan Research Division, she served for five decades, driving research into the chemical components that make infants develop normally, and dispelling the haze of rumour and half-practice that dominated paediatric practice previously.

Not surprisingly, much of her research focused on the composition of breast milk to determine the links between the mother's nutritional needs and the infant's growth. At the start of her career, the most advanced facilities screened milk for twelve chemical factors. By the time her studies were in full swing, over 200 separate components had been identified and catalogued according to their changing concentration over the course of nursing.

She put definitively to rest a prevailing slice of wisdom about the superiority of Jersey over Holstein milk and, more importantly, carried out tests about how best to enrich milk with Vitamin D while also conducting studies about the optimal amount needed to prevent rickets without a toxic vitamin overdose. If Vitamin D milk is a commonplace now, while rickets, once the scourge of America's slums, is not, much of the thanks for that must go to Macy.

But maybe it takes more to impress you than the eradication of a disease that grotesquely twisted the development of thousands of children annually. Very well, then. Macy's studies of the effects of deficiency of all vitamins led directly to the development of nutritive supplements for the children of low-income families that all but eliminated scurvy as well (some parents chose to use their children's lemon allotment to flavour their cocktails, as it turned out, thus the 'all but'). Five hundred and fifty children over the course of her study received some 280 tons of milk, 28 tons of vegetable soup, 5 tons of fruit, 2.5 tons of lemon juice powder/martini enhancer, and 300 gallons of cod liver oil (for its high Vitamin D content).

Her studies of the varying composition of blood during an infant's development led to the discovery of haemoglobin deficiency in many African American children, which in turn led to improved anaemia-screening practices; while her studies of breast milk determined that, although a mother produces natural barriers to make sure her child does not receive toxic overdoses of vitamins, there are no such barriers for artificial chemicals or drugs. These studies then prepared the way for an appreciation of the unique health problems facing children of alcoholic or drug-addicted mothers.

And not only *all of that*, but she also established a correlation between access to pre-natal care and the subsequent health and growth of the baby, the statistics from which contributed to the push for universal access to such care regardless of ability to pay, which lowered the birth risks to both mother and child and made our world of regular pregnancy check-up screenings a reality.

Somewhere in the midst of those vital studies, she married Dr Raymond Hoobler. She was 46, and he was 66, and seems to have been something of the bland but prosperous George Babbitt type, but he treated her well enough and, most importantly, supported her fully in continuing her career. They lived happily through the five years they had together before his death. She never remarried but devoted herself increasingly to large-scale nutrition projects, including a trip to India where she records herself as being astounded to find that, yes, women of other faiths seemed to care about their children's health too. (Her unconscious assumption that virtue is a unique property of Christians is one of her memoir's less charming aspects.)

She began in a world that barely knew what milk was and ended by not only exhaustively analysing its shifting composition, and not only detailing the extent and limits of a mother's chemical barriers, but perfecting methods to produce milk that would eliminate one of childhood's most ghastly diseases. Her work made care of the mother from the onset of pregnancy a priority, and showed the impact of food and shock on a child's development, and her larger nutritional studies provided baselines for nutritive value that made governmental relief programmes for poor children a targeted force for large-scale good.

And yet, in spite of the massive boon her work was for civilisation, my guess is that most of us have not heard of Icie Macy Hoobler. Because she worked with children, and child nutrition is a part of 'women's science', and women's science somehow does not count. Like Ellen Swallow, she was a researcher whose impact was measured in the millions of lives her work saved and enriched rather than in acclaim, and for her, if not for our own sense of justice, that was enough.

Further Reading

Macy's autobiography, *Boundless Horizons: Portrait of a Pioneer Woman Scientist* (1982), when it is not talking about Christians being necessarily virtuous and non-Christians as being surprisingly virtuous, is a charming delight. It is basically *Little House in the Big Woods* if Laura ended up becoming a kick-ass biochemist.

Chapter 24

War, Fame and Surgery

The Amazing Life of Margaret Chung, the First American-Born Chinese Woman Surgeon

Her mother was raised in a brothel, and her son was Ronald Reagan.

Take any section of Dr Margaret Chung's (1889–1959) life, and lay it against any other, and it is hard to believe they come from the biography of the same person. From an immigrant's daughter hauling vegetables to earn enough to eat, she ended life as a celebrity surgeon and wartime hero with a small army of adopted sons that included admirals, senators, actors and artists. A conservative Bohemian, a platonic lesbian, and a traditional modernist, Chung was a nexus of contradiction held together by will and grit, a woman out of her own time and yet who could have been produced by none other.

Chung's parents were immigrants from China who fell into the clutches of the late nineteenth-century American missionary system's benevolent despotism. A number of religious sects at the time looked at the misery of the Chinese immigrant community and realised with a sort of reptilian cunning that here lay opportunity. The Presbyterian Church in particular explicitly formed a strategy targeting young girls, theorising that a converted girl indoctrinated into a cult of motherhood and Christ would in turn be a centre of Christian conversion in her community, a community otherwise inaccessible to white missionaries.

Chung's parents were harvested by the Presbyterians in this manner under the public banner of charity and the private justification of sectarian tactics. Her mother, Lai Wan, was pulled at a young age from a brothel where she was working and given a home and stability in exchange for allowing herself to be made into the willing tool of the California Presbyterian Church's conversion strategy. Chung's father was similarly brought up through the Presbyterian ranks in a different city, attaining a reputation for unique devotion. The Church decided it would be advantageous to marry their two star creations off to each other, and they were duly thrown into each other's paths.

While this system of preying on immigrants' misery to create strongholds of religious belief in an otherwise inaccessible culture is transparently heinous to us now, at the time it was considered the height of charity, something you could never be thankful enough for having inflicted upon you. Chung's parents were lifelong attendees of their Church, and they passed their imposed modern Western Christian perspective on to the gaggle of seven children (out of *eleven* births) that they had been taught to produce by an iron doctrine of Tactical Fecundity encased in the velvet glove of Traditional Motherhood.

The serial births that Chung's mother endured in the name of that philosophy combined with tuberculosis to prematurely end her life, and much of the care for her enfeebled and worn body but persevering spirit fell to young Margaret. Her father kept the family moving as he started and failed in venture after venture, desperately trying to feed his large family via the handful of professions allowed a Chinese man in the late nineteenth century: raising and selling vegetables; agricultural labour; and the selling of 'traditional' Chinese items.

Margaret tended to her mother, went to school when she could, and worked every other moment to try and keep the family afloat, all the while guided by an ambition to become what the Presbyterian Church had taught her family was the noblest profession of all: a medical missionary. To young Margaret, it represented a chance to travel to a native land she had never seen and help those crippled by disease, and to the Church it was a golden opportunity to use foreign hospitals as potential conversion centres. Church circulars consequently lionised the profession. Margaret was resolute – a doctor she would be.

Women in the medical profession were, by this point, nowhere near as rare as even three decades before. Several of the schools that had opened mid-century to provide medical training for women had already folded, their boards determining that they were no longer needed with so many first rank co-educational medical colleges available. In 1907, Chung entered the USC Preparatory Academy, a high school that had connections to the USC College of Physicians and Surgeons. Graduates from the preparatory school could attend the college, meaning that Chung could go to medical school straight from high school, a situation common enough at the close of the nineteenth century but that was increasingly rare in the professionalised medical atmosphere of the early twentieth century.

Entering the College of Physicians and Surgeons in 1911, Chung began adopting the dress and mannerisms of the predominantly male colleagues around her, creating a persona she named 'Mike', sporting pulled-back hair and a man's sport jacket, and cultivating a taste for swearing, hunting and bawdy humour. Graduating from USC in 1916, she instantly applied for a position as a medical missionary to China, only to be peremptorily rejected.

Stunned by the rejection, Chung set about finding a new direction in life, working as a virtually unpaid surgeon in Chicago, as a psychological evaluator at a juvenile detention facility, and finally as a surgeon for the Santa Fe Railroad, where she developed a reputation for treating the company's Mexican workers with a compassion they were unaccustomed to receiving from the rest of the staff. She also slowly created a practice treating travelling performers and Hollywood professionals who would be critical to the establishment of her famous practice in San Francisco.

She fell in love with that city on a visit in the early 1920s and in 1922 decided to relocate her practice there, settling into the heart of Chinatown and revelling in the Bohemian delights of Nob Hill and Little Italy, exploring the romantic attraction to women that she felt, but which was condemned both by the religion she grew up in and the traditional Chinese community she was living among. As an unmarried, unconventional professional woman, her activities and Western leanings were viewed with distrust among the residents of Chinatown, even as her client base among the city's white population swelled.

Decking her office out in traditional Chinese trappings, Chung's practice was a cult destination for those seeking the benefits of Western medicine among the lush trappings of the exotic Orient. She was also known as one of the few doctors in the city willing to lend a compassionate ear to women seeking birth control and abortion, routinely referring such cases to doctors she knew to be professional and discreet. By 1931, Chung had established a routine that appeared glamorous from the outside but that she felt was personally unfulfilling: a thriving practice; proximity to the Bohemian and queer friendly nightlife of San Francisco; and a degree of material prosperity beyond the dreams of her hard scrabble childhood.

That year, however, her life was upturned when Japan invaded Manchuria and an unemployed pilot sought Chung out to ask her how he might volunteer his services in the defence of China. She had no connections with the Chinese military to speak of, but what she could do was cook him a nice meal and listen to his problems as a pilot in the depths of the Depression. Soon not only he, but his other pilot friends as well, made a ritual of taking dinner with Dr Chung. One fateful night they joked that they'd like to adopt her as their mother but were worried about lacking a father as a result. She fired back, calling them her Fair-Haired Bastards, and a legend was born.

The order of the Fair-Haired Bastards was duly founded, an ever-growing collection of pilots who met at 'Mom' Chung's once a week to eat a full meal, make connections, and hear her exhortations to get revenge on the Japanese invaders of her parents' native land. Over the 1930s, the association grew as Chung adopted thousands of pilots, submariners, admirals, and eventually celebrities (including a young Ronald Reagan) and congressmen. She was personally responsible for covertly drafting over 100 pilots to serve in the famous Flying Tigers squadron that served in China before America's entry into the Second World War.

With the entry of the United States into the war in 1941, Chung was launched from the realm of local curiosity to that of national celebrity. She became a potent symbol of Chinese–American cooperation to a nation that tended to lump the Chinese and Japanese together in one tangled lump of Otherness. The thousands of care packages she personally packed to send off to her sons overseas became the stuff of newspaper articles and even comic book features, and her web of military and governmental connections gave her a lobbying power unavailable to most Americans, let alone women of Chinese descent.

At the war's beginning, she parlayed that influence into momentum for the creation of a new military volunteer organisation, known to history as the WAVES. Though primarily associated with the name of its first director, Mildred McAfee, it was Chung who first proposed the idea of a naval branch for women, and collected enough political support to see that idea through the House and Senate. She expected to subsequently serve in the organisation that she had spearheaded, only to find her applications mysteriously rejected, perhaps because of rumours about her sexuality, perhaps simply because of her age (she was over 50 by the time of the organisation's founding).

Chung threw her time into the war effort, speaking where she could, tending to the injuries of returned adopted sons, raising money for the support of China, and writing thousands of letters to her boys on the front lines who otherwise would have received none. Her medical practice suffered as a result, and by war's end she was on the verge of having to give up her home when the Fair-Haired Bastards heard about it and raised money among themselves to pay her mortgage.

The war's end was the summit of Chung's hopes and the culmination of a decade and a half of behind-the-scenes support work, all carried off at the expense of her career as surgeon and physician. The next fourteen years saw her grow physically more frail, only able to work a couple of hours each day, while she threw herself into an intense but platonic relationship with singer-actress Sophie Tucker. The Chinese background that had led to the success of her practice and catapulted her to fame during the war worked increasingly against her over the 1950s, as Americans viewed China as another arm of the great Red Terror, and viewed with menace what they once found bursting with sumptuous exotic charm. She wrote an autobiography that would have been a best seller in 1944, but could not even find a publisher in the hardened climate of the 1950s.

Dr Margaret 'Mom' Chung underwent surgery for ovarian cancer in 1958 and, realising that the end could not be far off, set about putting her affairs in order, including plans for a funeral that would be as much a tribute to the thousands of adopted sons who had taken comfort in her words and acts of kindness as a summation of her life. She died on 5 January 1959. Her casket was borne to its final resting place by the mayor of San Francisco, two admirals of the navy, two privates and an ensign.

Further Reading

The story of Dr Chung's life was exhaustively researched and brought to light by the efforts of Judy Tzu-Chun Wu, whose 2005 *Doctor Mom Chung of the Fair-Haired Bastards: The Life of a Wartime Celebrity* is a powerful telling of the hardships faced by Chung's parents, and the improbably potent bond between Chung and her thousands of adopted sons. Like a lot of writing brought forth from the academic system, it tends to repeat its theses over and over again with slightly different wording, but the attraction of the story, and Wu's incredible work unearthing Chung's unpublished autobiography and hunting down surviving Fair-Haired Bastards more than compensates.

Chapter 25

Sex After Sixty

The Geriatric Gynaecology of Anna Kleegman Daniels

Sex after menopause. Drug addiction. Abortion.

In the early to mid-twentieth century, to be seen as casting an understanding eye on any one of these was to invite social ostracism. To crusade for enlightened attitudes towards these issues could be the work of a lifetime as you fought against the common wisdom that older women should simply stop having sex and graciously make way for their husbands' affairs, that the only way to deal with a drug addict was through state-orchestrated brutality, and that serial pregnancy unto death was the just wish of an all-knowing deity.

Being a social crusader on any of these fronts was a hard life. Being a social crusader for all three, well, that took a special sort of person, forged in hardship, and gifted with an indomitable optimism that empathy and understanding must ultimately win out over dogma and the red-limbed thirst for punishment. Fortunately for the people of the United States of America, a 12-year-old Ukrainian Jewish girl named Anna Kleegman (1893–1970) washed upon its shores with her pogrom-fleeing family in 1906 with the resolve already in her heart to dedicate her life to finding and alleviating suffering wherever she found it.

At every stage of her story, Kleegman showed super-human character and resolution, and never so much as in her early youth. Living in the Jewish ghetto of the small village of Borschevka, her father a revered rabbi and her mother a practical doer of deeds who had to work twice as hard to feed her family in light of her husband's Talmudic ethereality, the boundaries of Kleegman's life ought to have been tightly drawn: a minimal education; a well-arranged marriage; hiding in the forests from time to time to escape the worst of the tsar's pogroms; and a respectable death after a life of efficient housekeeping.

But Kleegman seized the wheel of her fate at the age of 5 and held on with white-knuckled intensity the rest of her life. At just 3 years old, she astounded the villagers with her ability to make exact change in her mother's small store. One of the entertainments of the ghetto was, in fact, to bring large bills to the store, make complicated purchases, and then watch this child prodigy produce the required change flawlessly.

At 5, Kleegman realised that, if she wanted to learn, *really* learn, about the world and its workings, she would need to go to the village's Russian school. Her father objected instantly and categorically. The Russian school met on Saturdays, and to learn on Saturday would be to break the Sabbath. The school had never accepted a Jewish student before, and certainly never a Jewish girl. It was impossible, ridiculous.

But Kleegman was not one to back down from something merely impossible. She learned Russian from her mother's customers until she could tell Krylov fables with dramatic perfection, and prevailed upon her father over and over again to give her the chance to learn. Eventually, the wise rabbi relented and obtained permission from the town council to allow Anna to attend the school's entrance examinations. She did, and performed so well that the school made an exception to admit her to its rolls.

There were two problems, however. Her family's poverty, and the matter of the Sabbath. But Anna knew precisely what to do. This now 6-year-old girl marched up to the school alone, asked the way to the school director's office in her newly learned peasant Russian, and let him know how it was going to be. Her family was too poor to pay, and she would have to be excused on Saturdays with the promise that she would do all the make-up work on Sunday. The director looked down at this indomitable girl and bowed before her superior force – the fee was waived, the absences allowed. Anna would go to school.

While there, she went from triumph to triumph, routinely the top student in her class, her only competition the brilliant son of the village mayor, who became her best friend and who begged his father to step in and sign her valedictorian certificate when the village priest refused to do so (it would be an affront to God, after all, to certify a Jewish girl as the smartest in her class). Having gone as far as she could in her country, she turned her eyes to a land that not only educated women, but allowed them to become professors and doctors: The United States.

Her father at first did not want to go. He had a respectable intellectual position in a traditional community and could not reconcile himself to taking up a new life in an electric world. But world events conspired to change the rabbi's mind. Antisemitic pogroms were intensifying all throughout the tsar's dominions, even to the extent of encompassing as small an enclave of Jewish life as the Borschevka ghetto. The family were driven from their home once, clutching one of Anna's fever-ridden sisters in a pile of blankets as they did so, to hide in the woods while Christians savaged their home, and there was no evidence of things getting better soon.

Meanwhile, Russia had stumbled into war with Japan, and further into the maddening embarrassment of losing that war. The mangled farm sons who had been conscripted into the tsar's army started returning home, limbs lost, wounds open, too poor to call for a doctor, and entirely forgotten by the army that had used them, broken them, and then let them loose to survive as best they could. Anna's mother saw the parade of suffering and resolved to do something. She tore up her wedding dress to make bandages and took her daughter into the fields to find the herbs required for healing salves and then, her young daughter in tow, strapped some old sacks on their feet by way of shoes and started walking from village to village in search of wounded soldiers to help.

'The world is filled with people who do nothing, who let terrible things happen and are only glad it isn't happening to them,' her mother said as they made their trek and the bags binding their feet disintegrated under them, 'That's no way to live in the world. You must behave as though everything you do is important; then it will be.'

At the trip's end, Anna turned to her mother and said,

> Mother, when we go to America, I won't be a teacher; all a teacher can do is tell people things – wonderful things and important things. But you are right it is not enough to tell people. You must do. People only really understand what you do. There are not enough doctors in Russia for the people. I will learn to be a doctor, and then I will come back here and treat the peasants.

Young Anna had her next goal in sight and, as before, it was up to the world to get out of her way. The family emigrated in 1906 and, according to the educational structure of the time, Anna had to be knocked back down to first grade because she knew no English. The prodigy was now the awkward oldest child in the class, but of course she would not allow herself to remain in that position. In a matter of five months, she worked herself up from grade 1 to grade 8, driving herself to learn unaccented English so that she could get on to her real work. She then graduated from high school in two years and, lying about her age just a smidge, went to Cornell University on a scholarship at age 15.

From that moment, Kleegman was a medical force sweeping all opposition before her. There were some perfunctory efforts by professors and doctors to keep her from various appointments or from talking about certain subjects, but how could those paper soldiers hope to stand long before the indomitable will of Battleship Kleegman? She quickly became one of the great Characters of New York City life. It is deeply tempting to fill this entire appreciation of her life with Kleegman anecdotes, stories of how she would always arrive to formal dinners three hours late with four or five strangers she met along the way straggling behind her; how she drove a two-seat Whippet and would stuff pedestrians who looked as though they could use a lift on top of each other in the second seat, in the trunk, and on the hood, to help them get a bit further up the road; or how she would shanghai friends with the promise of a bracing swim at her beach house only to lead them on a five-hour long goose chase through errands she had to run, ending in a freezing dash to a rain-soaked beach and the promise of sleep in a bungalow without a roof.

Her private life was the real-world incarnation of Katherine Hepburn's character in *Bringing Up Baby* – a swirling vortex of chaos that threatened to suck everybody in its radius into an unintended and maddening adventure, smoothed over by the absolute purity of her intentions. But we are here to celebrate Dr Anna Kleegman Daniels, the physician, and so it is high time to get down to the matter of the work she won fame for.

She did not go back to Russia to tend the peasants, as there was a sufficiency of suffering right in her neighbourhood to fill a lifetime. She became a physician, concentrating increasingly on work as an obstetrician and gynaecologist. With her sister, Sophia Kleegman, she was an early advocate for birth control and sex education. Faced with the steady parade of broken and desperately poor women, terrified at the prospect of giving birth to another mouth they could not hope to feed, how could you not put your shoulder behind the effort to educate women about the workings of their own bodies, and placing in their hands the ability to break the crushing cycle of serial pregnancy thrust upon them by religion and tradition?

To those who were at the last step of desperation, seeking an illegal abortion, Kleegman's first instinct was invariably to fix the circumstances that underpinned that desperation. If husbands were unemployed, she would make a call and find them work. If they did not have room for more children, she would make another call and find a better living space at a lower rate. But if, for all that, the mother was still determined that this child could only know suffering, Kleegman would direct them to a responsible physician to perform an abortion. She refused to carry out the policy herself, but she would not allow a desperate woman to run into the arms of a back-alley surgeon, and soon Dr Kleegman was recognised as a doctor who listened, and understood.

It is the middle part of Kleegman's career that we know the best, however, as an author of books and articles about the biology of the post-menopausal woman. Historically in Western culture, menopause was the sharp break between Woman the Sexual-Reproductive Object, to be sought after and captured and Woman the, Well, We're Really Not Quite Sure, but definitely NOT Sexual Object. Julian Haubold-Stolle's book *Oma ist die Beste* (2009) documents the ins and outs of how elderly women have been viewed in Western society, originating in a fear that manifested itself in the witch or hag topos. Here, old women are forces of evil who seek to leech fertility from the young – sinister presences to be avoided. Of course, every thesis has its antithesis, and when the pendulum next swung it was all the way to the side of the Beatific Victorian Grandmother, the baker of cookies and sewer of quilts who was so de-sexualised that she could not even possibly be conceived of as a threat.

Synthesis came in the form of Dr Anna Kleegman Daniels, whose book *It's Never Too Late to Love* (1953) argued strenuously for the continued sexuality of women post-menopause. It was shocking, even more shocking somehow than her espousal of birth control and sex education. Grandfathers having a bit of a dalliance with the office secretary, certainly, and only natural, but grand*mothers*? An abomination! She gathered her considerable energies to do combat with the myths that led women into frustrated lives of seclusion:

> Thanks to our excessive prudishness and our lamentable habit of confusing ignorance with innocence, there is more misinformation, superstition and mystery about sex than about any other subject under the sun. This is not only a pity, but often a tragedy. For sex is an integral, vital part of every human being. As the result of centuries of old-wives' tales and dark, secret whisperings the menopause has become a grisly hobgoblin that has terrified countless generations of women. Around this most normal physical function have clustered a small army of myths like moths around a flame.

She combined her gynaecology practice with marriage counselling to advise women about the physical realities and potentials of their new lives, and to counsel men and women together about what to expect, how to help each other, and most importantly, what they could look forward to.

By the 1960s, the girl who had come to America fleeing the pogroms of tsarist Russia was an old woman looking out at a world bristling with radically new social challenges. But the youth movement of the 1960s, that caused many educated persons of her generation to retrench into a dispirited conservatism, saw Kleegman extending her broad-minded empathy even further than she had in her youth. She saw everywhere around her young people felled by drug addiction, and a justice system more intent on punishing than healing them, and knew instinctively that here was a cause to which she could give the last years of her life.

Throughout her late sixties and early seventies, she moved away from marriage counselling and towards developing therapies that weaned drug addicts from their addictions. In spite of being held at knifepoint and gunpoint by addicts demanding that she supply them with addictive medications, she continued her practice, meeting her patients alone and unarmed in spite of her family's vigorous requests to find a less dangerous group of patients.

They should have known better. She had stared down a school administrator at 6, the medical establishment at 20, and now at 70 she was hardly likely to back down from helping those who lived at the tottering edges of the medical and penal systems' organised ire. She continued faithfully serving the Forgotten of her adopted country until her sudden death in 1970.

Further Reading

My Mother, the Doctor (1970), written by Anna's daughter Joy Daniels, is delightful in every aspect. There is not that much on her scientific contributions there, but as a sketch of an Auntie Mame-like medical crusader, it is absolutely irresistible. Kleegman also wrote a book about the sexual life of post-menopausal women, *It's Never Too Late to Love*, which is a classic of which some parts have aged better than others.

Chapter 26

Blue Babies with Crossword Puzzle Hearts

The Paediatric Cardiology of Helen Taussig

It is sometime in the 1930s, and you are walking into a ward full of crouching children with blue-tinted lips. Something is wrong with their hearts, something that is preventing their blood from getting enough oxygen, turning the red fluid a deep, thick black. At the slightest exertion, the children can pass out and even die, their starved tissues and thickening heart unable to cope with the effort. Next to them are the parents who have been told to expect the worst, and to expect it soon. They are 'blue babies', victims of a congenital heart defect for which nobody holds out any hope of a cure.

At this time in the history of medicine, the heart was a surgical Forbidden Zone where none but the bravest dared tread. Fortunately, for the tens of thousands that have been since cured of the heart condition that produces blue babies, an unlikely trio of medical legends arrived on the scene to change all that: Alfred Blalock, whose research on shock and crush syndrome would deserve him the thanks of humanity even if he had never operated on a single heart; Vivien Thomas, a surgical wizard who was kept from title and decent pay most of his career by virtue of his skin colour; and our subject today, paediatric cardiologist Helen Taussig (1898–1986).

Taussig's mother, Edith Guild Taussig, was a remarkable person. She was a graduate of Radcliffe in that institution's experimental first years, a student of biology and botany who communicated her enthusiasms to her daughter. For eleven years, Helen and Edith explored the outdoors and cultivated their garden, until Edith was taken away by tuberculosis and left the young Helen to be raised by her father, an economics professor who always supported her during the setbacks of her adolescent years.

And there were many. She found reading difficult, probably because of some form of dyslexia that her era was unequipped to recognise. When she went to college at Radcliffe, she felt that she was just the daughter of the great Professor Taussig rather than a human being in her own right, and so she transferred to Berkeley to finish her studies. She decided to go into public health, and went to Harvard to deepen her knowledge, where she was informed that she could take classes, but could never, as a woman, be awarded a degree. Infuriated by the administration's openly expressed disdain for female students, she attended classes anyway, only to find that she was made to sit apart from the rest of her classmates and, during laboratory work, was confined in a totally separate room.

Fortunately, one of her professors recommended she study instead at Boston University, where anatomy classes were open to women (which was decidedly *not* the case at Harvard). While there one day, an instructor tossed a cow heart into her hands and told her to study it. She delved into the intricacies of the heart with vigour, spending long nights studying the contractions of mammalian cardiac tissue.

She put in an application at Johns Hopkins, which as we will remember from Florence Sabin's story, was financed by grants from a group of women who had attached the acceptance of women as doctoral candidates as a condition of their financing. She was accepted in 1924 and given an internship in paediatrics to assist in the formation of the university's paediatric cardiac clinic. Things had been going so suddenly well that it was high time for life to send another delightful curve: in 1930, Taussig lost her hearing. She was a paediatric cardiologist who was robbed of the ability to listen to her patients' heartbeats, a bitter irony of Beethoven-esque proportions. Rather than giving up her hard-won position, however, she taught herself how to feel heartbeats with her hands and to employ fluoroscope technology to tell her what her hands could not reveal.

She began her work studying diseases that afflicted the heart, such as rheumatic fever, but was soon nudged in the direction of congenital heart malformations, a career path that seemed a dead end at the time. After all, bacteria could be fought, but if a heart was malformed since birth, there was, at the time, nothing to be done. The major vessels around the heart were just starting to be talked of as likely objects of surgery, but the heart itself? Why study afflictions that had no possibility of remedy?

But when you are an intern, and you are told to study something, that is what you do. Taussig corresponded with Maude Abbott, a world expert on congenital heart problems, studied the patients in her ward, and soon found a link between a series of four defects called the tetralogy of Fallot and a condition known as Blue Baby Syndrome. In tetralogy patients, the pulmonary artery is constricted, meaning that less blood makes it from the heart to the lungs for oxygenation. As a result, the right ventricle has to pump harder than usual, thickening its walls. At the same time, there is a hole connecting the two ventricles that really ought not be there, and a displacement of the aorta, both of which allow deoxygenated blood from the right ventricle to sneak over into the left ventricle for shipment throughout the body.

Children with this constellation of defects have an understandably low oxygen count in their blood, rendering it thick and nearly black, causing the tell-tale bluish complexion that gives the condition its name. It also means that tissues wear out fast, unable to supply themselves with enough oxygen from the blood to maintain any extended exertion. Historically, children with the condition invariably died young.

There was not much to do but keep patients comfortable and relaxed, until 1939 when Taussig heard about an operation performed by Robert Gross. He had successfully performed a surgery to close off a *ductus arteriosus*, a blood vessel that links the pulmonary arteries to the aorta. For foetuses, it is a useful vessel. We get all our oxygen from our mother, so having a duct that moves blood straight back into the aorta, bypassing the lungs, is not a bad idea. After birth, this duct is supposed to close up again, allowing blood to flow from the arteries to the lungs, and then back to the heart for distribution through the aorta.

Taussig realised that the *ductus arteriosus* was the answer to her problem. If a duct could be safely closed surgically, why could not one be *added*? That would provide a second pathway for blood to get to the lungs, bypassing the narrowed pulmonary arteries. If it could be done, it could provide a way for blood to obtain a normal amount of oxygen, and cure the children in her ward. She brought the idea to Gross, who couldn't understand why you would want to insert the very duct he had just become famous for sewing up.

He was not helpful. But the next people she brought the idea to were. There are conflicting accounts about just how Vivien Thomas, Alfred Blalock and Helen Taussig developed the operation that cured blue babies, but it seems to be a case of marvellous serendipity. Blalock and Thomas had been working on techniques to join blood vessels on to each other, and Taussig had an idea for relieving the blue baby symptoms through joining the aorta and the pulmonary artery. The actual surgery was performed in 1944 on a 15-month-old child named Eileen Saxon. Everything was set up to go wrong. All the experiments on dogs to refine the procedure had been performed by Vivien Thomas, but it was Blalock who was performing the first human surgery. The dog vessels they had been working with were twice the size of tiny Eileen's. All that everybody in the room knew was that, without the surgery, Eileen would die, and soon.

Blalock performed the surgery with Thomas standing behind him and Taussig watching nervously on. It was a success, as was the next surgery. The pink colour returned to Eileen's lips while she was still on the table. Taussig and Blalock were vaulted to celebrity status, while Thomas, the African American technician who had perfected the procedure, was pushed to the shadows of obscurity. John Hopkins was suddenly swamped with children from all over the world, their parents desperate for the emergency procedure. Blalock himself performed the surgery over a thousand times, while Taussig was responsible for diagnosing the patients and overseeing their treatment and recovery.

Through her research and persistence, Taussig had saved the lives of thousands of children. That's sufficient laurels for just about anybody, but Taussig was not done yet. She had one more service to offer us.

In the late 1950s and early 1960s, waves of children were being born throughout Europe with *phocomelia*, popularly known as Seal Limbs. These children had their hands and feet growing directly out of their torsos, a developmental problem coming from seemingly nowhere. She talked with Widukind Lenz, a German physician who was investigating the matter. His conclusion was that the defects were being caused by Contergan, the brand name of thalidomide, a sleeping medication that was considered so harmless it was sold over the counter. Lenz's results in hand, she returned to America, where thalidomide was being distributed to doctors even though it had not yet received FDA approval.

In this era before tightened federal regulation, it was a regular occurrence for pharmaceutical companies to offer medication directly to doctors before that medication was actually cleared by the government. Sixteen thousand people, and 200 pregnant mothers, had taken it under these loose conditions, a recipe for disaster that Taussig met head-on by publishing her findings in every scientific journal that would listen, and in speeches at the American College of Physicians and Johns Hopkins University. Thalidomide was pulled from production and every hospital that had received samples was tracked down and their supplies recovered. As a result, while Europe and Africa witnessed 10,000 seal baby births, the United States only had 17. Not only that, but the scrutiny Taussig had shone upon the practices of the pharmaceutical industry caused President Kennedy to enact new legislation to tighten the FDA process.

Not bad, Dr Taussig.

Taussig continued working with children and their 'crossword problem' hearts, writing a third of her scientific papers *after* having supposedly retired. She lived to see one of the blue babies her surgery had saved give a virtuoso piano recital in her honour; to win the Kober Medal and serve as the first woman president of the American Heart Association.

Helen Taussig died in 1986 in an automobile crash.

Further Reading

In spite of the importance of her work, there is no full-length adult biographical treatment of her life. Lisa Yount's *Mending Children's Hearts: Alfred Blalock, Helen Taussig & Vivien Thomas* is a middle- to high-school level book that is about your best bet. Vivien Thomas also wrote a memoir, but it is *not* for the weak of stomach. He describes the often-grizzly surgical procedures of Blalock's research laboratory in minute detail and, if you are squeamish like me, that makes it a hard book to get through, though fascinating. There is also a movie about the events surrounding the blue baby surgery starring none other than the late Alan Rickman and Mos Def, *Something the Lord Made*. It is a good film, but Taussig's role in suggesting the basic mechanism of the surgery is transferred entirely to Blalock and Thomas, reducing Taussig to basically That Female Doctor That Works With Kids And Has A Problem It's Up to Us Brilliant Men To Fix. Still, Mos Def is astounding in it, so it is worth watching.

Chapter 27

Making All Nurses Equal

The Many Battles of Estelle Massey Osborne

In 1923, when Estelle Massey graduated from the City Hospital No. 2 School of Nursing with the highest examination score in the entire state of Missouri, only fourteen of the nation's 1,300 schools for nursing allowed black people to even apply. The American Nurses Association did not accept black nurses as members, and the US navy categorically refused to employ them. And while it is an oversimplification to attribute the opening of the nursing profession to minorities throughout the 1950s and 1960s to a single person, it was assuredly the multi-front plan formed by Estelle Massey (1901–1981) while president of the National Association of Colored Graduate Nurses that provided the blueprint for overcoming the worst of the profession's inequalities.

Estelle Massey invented no new medical technique – the time she spent as an actual practising nurse was far outweighed by her time as an administrator and organiser – and because our society is as it is, you have probably never heard of her. We lionise doctors, but tend towards condescension when it comes to nurses; we celebrate researchers but mock administrators. And yet it was this tireless nurse-turned-administrator who did the long, hard work of erecting new educational institutions for black nurses and forging relations with theretofore white-exclusive national organisations that, after persistent decades, at last stamped out one of the great prejudices at the heart of the American health system. For all that, she deserves far more than the smattering of thin articles she has been allotted by historians of science.

She was born the eighth of eleven children in the small town of Palestine, Texas. Her parents believed resolutely in the power of education, and all of Massey's older sisters became teachers. Her mother had two principles in raising her daughters – that they must complete high school and that they must never, so long as they were children, work for white people. She wanted to shield her daughters from the indignities of prejudice for as long as possible; to let them grow into a confident sense of identity before subjecting them to the self-shattering blows of white objectification.

By and large, she succeeded. With the exception of a white police officer who propositioned her, at the age of 11, to let him buy her a pair of shoes she was looking at in a window in exchange for sexual favours, she grew up without the daily indignities of segregated transportation and dehumanisation at the hands of white employers. She graduated high school and, as had her sisters before her, set out at age 18 to her first teaching position.

She was the only teacher at a school for farmers' children where all children were piled in one room regardless of age, the sort of set-up we associate with the mid-1800s but that, along the periphery of American education, was still very much in existence into the 1920s.

It was not Massey's thing. Parents pulled their children from class for most of the year to help with the harvest, and the town itself offered no stimulation for a bright young woman used to the lively intellectual atmosphere of her parents' home. When a man at the school was mysteriously killed by a gunshot through the classroom window, Massey took it as an unambiguous sign to 'get out of Dodge' and resigned her post.

She went to live with her brother, a dentist in St Louis, with the idea of taking up dentistry herself. Her brother, however, did not think it was the right fit for her and conspired with some friends to lure her into the nearby hospital's new nurse training programme. They were taking Basically Anybody, and when she turned up to get a feel for the place she found to her surprise, and warranted concern, that she was immediately accepted into the programme. Before she quite realised what had happened, she found herself studying nursing and developing a genuine passion for it, particularly obstetrics.

She studied for three years, obtained the highest score on the state-wide final nurse's exam, and, given her love of obstetrics, was of course immediately placed in a position that had nothing to do with obstetrics. The theory at the time was that, to develop discipline in a new nurse, you had to place them in a position they were actively not passionate about. Massey was stuck at the medical ward, checking patients in and out – routine work that was in no way satisfying – so when an opportunity arose to work in public health, she grabbed it, taking a job with the Municipal Visiting Nurses of St Louis, where she was assigned the cases involving minorities.

Here she came up against the real dead weight of institutional prejudice. When her superiors vacated their positions, their jobs went to other white people of less seniority and training than Massey, and when official calls came in, the callers routinely insisted on talking to the white nurses, even if it was about topics in Massey's area of experience. As a result, sometimes

Massey would answer the phone, be forced to hand it to a nearby white nurse, but then sit close by as that white nurse relayed questions from the caller to her, and her responses back to the caller, in a hurtful farce.

So, she left that position too, heading for work at a joint programme between a Kansas City high school, junior college and a couple of local hospitals to exchange educational opportunities. She taught nursing and hygiene at the high school and college, but felt that, to do her job properly, she ought to have more education herself than three years at the world's least picky nursing programme. She applied for a Rosenwald Fund scholarship even though one had never been given to a black nursing student before, and boldly resigned her post before hearing that she had won it.

Fortunately, she did, and in 1931, she became the first black nurse ever to earn a master's degree. She was selected by the Rosenwald Fund to apply her new learning to a project in the deep South, investigating ways to bring better health education and service to rural communities. As might be imagined, a young black professional showing up in the South and advising white townsmen about health initiatives often sparked resentment. One official told her not to appoint any nurses who gave black people too much respect by saying 'Mr' or 'Mrs' in front of their last names. She learned to navigate prejudice with cool detachment, while at the same time discovering that allies often were found in unlikely places. That knowledge served her well in her next position, as she stepped on to a truly national stage.

She took up the educational directorship of Freedmen's Hospital in DC (another first for a black woman) and soon the presidency of the National Association of Colored Graduate Nurses (NACGN), a position she held for five years, from 1934 to 1939. During her tenure, she unleashed a two-pronged assault, firstly forming connections with the wider nursing community that paved the way for black nurses to be integrated into the American Nurses Association, and secondly by fostering programmes that developed post-nursing school opportunities for nurses of colour. By 1946, the ANA began its integration, and by 1951 the NACGN dissolved itself as no longer necessary in the face of the ANA's new inclusivity.

While the NACGN and ANA were working out the details of the project Massey had started, Massey herself had moved on in the early 1940s to a position at the National Nursing Council for War Service (yet another first), where she was tasked with investigating how black nurses could be incorporated at last into the armed services, in anticipation of the Second World War. At the time, in the army black nurses accounted for less than 0.5 per cent of the total, while there were precisely zero serving in the navy. Massey applied pressure on the armed forces to change their policies, and grouped together professional organisations to persuade educational institutions to allow nursing students of colour.

As a direct result, in just two years, the fourteen training schools available during Massey's youth shot up to thirty-eight, the number of minority army nurses in the army doubled, and the navy began allowing black nurses as well.

Four of them.

After the war, she joined the Board of Directors of the ANA (yet another first) and was sent to Sweden to represent America at the International Council of Nurses. Four years with the ANA (1948–1952) was followed by a long reign as assistant director of the National League for Nursing (1954–1959) followed by a position as the full Director of Services, where she continued to open the South and expand education.

She lived for twenty-one years after becoming director, but no account of her life during the years 1964–1981 exists, so what she did during that time, including even the circumstances of her death, remains a great unnecessary mystery, created by chroniclers of nursing's history simply losing interest in her story. The last source to devote more than a few paragraphs to her life came out in 1966, and all historians since have remained content to end their narratives there, in spite of access to records that might fill in those aching blanks.

And so, we say goodbye to Massey in 1965, at the height of her influence, and with the sincere hope that someone who meant so much to an oppressed minority in an under-appreciated profession had a peaceful end, replete with the full knowledge of all she had meant, to nursing, to people of colour, and indeed to the world.

Further Reading

The sources are, as I mentioned, depressing in their abrupt fall-off. The redoubtable Edna Yost gives her thirty-ish pages in *American Women of Nursing* (1947), and she also shows up for six pages in *The Story of Nursing* (1954, revised 1965) by Bertha Dodge. Those narratives get combined in your best source overall, the twelve over-sized pages devoted to Osborne in the nursing section of Volume 2 of *Profiles of Negro Womanhood* (1966), which is a great series by Sylvia Dannett for anybody interested in the history of black women in America.

Chapter 28

Isabel Morgan, Polio, and the High Cost of Marriage

Polio, unique among humanity's eradicated diseases, carries with it a visual familiarity that has insistently lingered far beyond its demise:

- Boys and girls with leg braces and dual crutches.
- FDR in his wheelchair.
- Rooms full of iron lungs mechanically keeping children alive.

Paradoxically, that very familiarity has defanged our towering horror of the disease somewhat – we realise that all of these are terrible things, but they do not seem quite real precisely because we have such a firm grip on the peripherals and paraphernalia involved. It is not until you sink into the personal stories of the era that the clawing helplessness polio left in its wake comes staggeringly alive again.

Stories of families living in perfect happiness until one day a daughter complains of a stiff neck, and dies that night. And then another child the next. And another child the next. And another the next. We no longer have the visceral experience to understand that sheer, incomprehensible chasm of powerlessness in the face of a force that empties bed after bed in your house in spite of every effort, every sacrifice, you make to keep it at bay. Polio actually did not kill that many people compared to, say, the great influenza epidemic, but its ability to reach precisely those families that considered themselves the safest and cut them down put every family in a state of omnipresent fear stretching from the outbreak of the epidemic in 1916 until the late 1950s.

Jonas Salk was lauded as a hero, and rightfully so, when he unveiled his killed-virus vaccine in a sweeping series of tests in 1954, but for thousands that was too late. Massive outbreaks of polio in the early 1950s had taken their toll, and there are those still suffering today who just might have avoided their fate had it not been for one man and one marriage.

Isabel Morgan (1911–1996) was scientific royalty. She was the daughter of Thomas Hunt Morgan (1866–1945), the Nobel Prize-winning biologist whose work with *Drosophila melanogaster* had laid out definitively the chromosomal foundations of heredity, and experimental biologist Lilian Sampson, and her mother home-schooled her up to the third grade. Of her early life, we know little until we find her graduating from Stanford University in the early 1930s. In 1936, she received her master's degree from Cornell, and in 1940 her doctoral thesis on *Histopathological Changes Produced in Rabbits by Experimental Inoculation with Hemolytic Streptococci and Certain of their Component Factors* was accepted at the University of Pennsylvania.

By 1938, she was at the Rockefeller Institute for Medical Research, performing research on polio and encephalomyelitis that garnered for her a position at Johns Hopkins, where David Bodian and Howard Howe were working on categorising the serotypes, or varieties, of poliovirus that existed. Attempts to craft vaccines up to that point had largely worked on the assumption that there was only one primary variety, and as a result were ineffective. Morgan found that there were in fact three distinct serotypes, which would all have to be taken into account to produce a successful vaccine.

From 1944 to 1949 she also worked on the problem of how to create a polio vaccine that used killed viruses to trigger our immunity mechanisms. If possible, this method had marked advantages over the use of weakened, living viruses. Killing viruses is easier than weakening them, and dead viruses do not spring back into virulence the same way that even the most skilfully weakened ones have a habit of doing. The problem was that in the 1930s a scientist named Maurice Brodie had claimed he had used killed viruses to trigger the production of antibodies, but nobody was able to replicate his results, and as a result by the 1940s the virological community had largely abandoned killed viruses as a stimulant to the immune system.

But then, in 1949, Morgan crafted a batch of dead viruses grown in the neural tissue of a monkey, and injected it into another animal. The theory was that the infusion of dead viruses would jog the immune system to create antibodies which it could use to fight off future attacks of polio. The crucial test came when she injected very much alive polio directly into that monkey's brain and waited to see if it would come down with polio. It did not. The principle of the killed-virus vaccine had been proven. Morgan then went one step further – showing why perhaps Brodie's results had been difficult to replicate – by demonstrating that killed-virus vaccines worked best when given as a series of injections, which early researchers had not attempted, an idea which forms the basis of our modern, and by now very familiar, practice of employing booster shots.

All was going well, and then a man named Joseph Mountain came along and asked Isabel to marry him, and she did, dropping her research to start a life with him in Westchester, caring for his handicapped child of a former marriage and his household while taking what satisfaction she could in the lesser scientific facilities available to her at Westchester County's Department of Laboratory Research. Whether because she balked at the dangers inherent in pushing her polio research into the next stage, which would have involved human testing, or because her new department lacked the resources that had been available to her at Johns Hopkins, she gave up her polio work, and by 1960 had switched to biostatistics as her field of study, carrying out epidemiological studies of the health impacts of air pollution.

Nobody at Johns Hopkins picked up her work, and the killed-virus vaccine had to wait for another six years before Salk was able to come up with his own version and distribute it widely. In the interim, two disastrous years of outbreak had left thousands of children dead. To be fair, some of the breakthroughs that Salk required, and that Morgan would have needed before mass-producing a safe and effective vaccine, were not available in 1949. Dorothy Horstmann's discovery that polio multiplied in the small intestine, and so could be fought in the bloodstream, opened the way for new and safer approaches to vaccine delivery and replication that Morgan would have either had to discover for herself, or to wait until 1952 to read about in Horstmann's paper like everybody else, but the general consensus seems to be that her work was a solid year ahead of Salk's, and in epidemiology a year of uncontrolled outbreak can be a massive and terrifying thing.

The last part of Morgan's career concentrated on studies of cancer therapies, work that she continued until 1979. She passed away in Arlington, Virginia in 1996.

Further Reading

Because Morgan's career was cut short, you will pretty much only find her in larger books about polio, of which a deservedly revered one is David Oshinsky's *Polio: An American Story* (2005). It covers both the medical end, with stories of Salk and Sabin, Horstmann and Morgan, and the truly massive public relations machinery engineered by the March of Dimes to fund the drive for a vaccine, so there is something in there for everybody.

Chapter 29

Killer of Cancer, Slayer of Viruses

The Many Medicines of Nobel Prize Laureate Gertrude Elion

Generally, our experience of a particular medicine is as a great faceless thing the name of which we do not know until we desperately need it, and the creation of which we assume is the end product of some unknowable corporate mixture of dark wizardry and exquisite micro pipetting. 'Who made this?' rarely crosses our minds, much less, 'What did they sacrifice so that I might benefit from it now?'

Were we slightly more curious about these matters, we might find that a good number of the medications that save members of our species thousands of times over on a daily basis have their root in one remarkable human being: Nobel Prize winner Gertrude Elion (1918–1999). Her mind and approach to medical invention generated not only the first medication effective against leukaemia, but the first immuno-suppressing drug that allowed for organ transplants, the first drug to be effective against a virus, and an array of other compounds that fought (and continue to fight) gout, lupus, herpes, malaria and sepsis.

Her contribution to the betterment of human existence is truly incalculable, which is all the more amazing considering her late entry into pharmaceutical research. The daughter of Jewish immigrant parents, she grew up in an atmosphere where her love of learning and tendency to lionise the great scientific minds of the past were fostered and encouraged. She read Paul de Kruif's *Microbe Hunters*, the 1926 classic that likewise inspired Jonas Salk in his choice of career, and knew that she wanted to find something new that might help people.

Her problem, however, was that of many talented young polymaths. Where ought she to concentrate her talents? She was just as quick at study of languages and history as she was of the natural sciences, and did not feel a definitive pull in any particular direction until her grandfather, whose attention and support had been so important to her as a child, fell ill with stomach cancer. At the time, she was a student at the City College of New York, which she had chosen because it was free and her family's finances were all but wiped out during the Great Depression. She decided that chemistry, and in particular the connection between chemistry and disease, would be the main thrust of her life's work.

Graduating in 1937 with highest honours, Elion set about the task of finding meaningful employment as a budding chemist during the long-lingering Depression, only to find all doors closed, not because no jobs were available but because no jobs were available for a *woman* chemist. As a result, one of the greatest scientific minds of her generation was compelled to fritter away seven long years in a series of secretarial, substitute teaching and flat-out temporary positions at anywhere that would take her. She did, however, manage to save up enough money as a result to attend graduate classes at New York University, gathering up the knowledge and experience that would prove essential when her nation was at last desperate enough to call upon her gifts.

The Second World War brought a whole new level of industrial-scale needs to the American landscape, needs which had to be filled by women if the requirements of intercontinental warfare were to be met. In such an atmosphere, it would have been odd for a single professional with Elion's credentials to remain unutilised, but for two years, until 1944, that is precisely what happened. She was given laboratory work, certainly, but not precisely research of the first rank. Her first job was as a food tester for A & P grocery stores, checking vanilla bean freshness and pickle acidity, among other similarly workaday tasks.

After two years of that work, in which she learned how to use a variety of instruments but little else, she found work at Johnson and Johnson, but when she was offered a position as a suture tensile strength tester, she refused. Time was slipping through her fingers – nearly a decade had passed since her graduation and she was nowhere near realising the dreams of her youth or the vows she made by her grandfather's deathbed.

A chance word from her father, however, placed her life suddenly on a brand-new trajectory. He was a dentist by trade, and one day he mentioned a company that had been sending him samples and which had a factory close to the family's New York residence. The company was Burroughs Wellcome, founded in England in 1880 with the mission of discovering new drugs in the fight against humanity's deadliest diseases. The company's goal was original research, run by scientists who were given free rein to investigate whatever interested them. Elion invited herself over for an interview, secured a job, and began working under a scientist by the name of George Hitchings.

Together, Hitchings and Elion would revolutionise how new medicines are discovered, though the relationship was not always smooth. Hitchings could be egotistical and harsh, but he was also willing to let Elion follow her own instincts, and to place her name first on the papers announcing her discoveries (certainly not a universal practice, especially as regards women subordinate scientists in the early twentieth century). Hitchings was frustrated with the traditional approach to medicinal discovery, the random combing through nature for compounds that might, or might not, do something to some disease somehow. He wanted a more rigorous, biochemical-based approach, which looked at the life cycle of a disease and its chemical stages and crafted medications that interfered with that cycle without simultaneously interfering with the functioning of a human's regular cells.

In Elion he found a perfect disciple, a scientist passionately and selflessly devoted to the eradication of disease, and willing to work appalling hours to determine the chemical cycles and metabolic processes of diseases in order to develop targeted medicines to combat them. He set her to work on purine research, which would dominate the first decades of her career. Purines and pyrimidines are the two types of bases that are found in RNA and DNA, and the cycle by which purines are degraded and recycled is central to the ability of any cell to function.

In the late 1940s, it was known that nucleic acids like DNA and RNA carried genetic information, and that purines and pyrimidines were important chemical components of nucleic acid structure, but that structure had yet to be fully elucidated by the work of Wilkins, Franklin, Watson and Crick in the 1950s. Elion's task, then, was to determine the important intermediate chemicals in the life cycle of a purine, and to attempt to develop compounds that were *like* those intermediate chemicals (or that broke down into such chemicals), but chemically useless. The idea was that if you could flood a harmful cell with useless but similar versions of a chemical it needed to function, then it might be tricked into using those chemicals in place of the functional varieties, and would as such not be able to synthesise the basic compounds it needed to survive.

This was the compelling kind of work that Elion had dreamed of since her childhood, and it would ultimately bear the most rewarding possible results, but before she crossed the threshold into her years as a mature scientist, one terrible trial awaited her. She had been working on her PhD at the Brooklyn Polytechnic Institute for a number of years while simultaneously carrying out her research at Burroughs Wellcome when she was summoned by the BPI dean and told that, if she wanted to keep pursuing her PhD, she would have to quit her job at Burroughs. She was faced with a terrible decision – continue towards her PhD but at the cost of abandoning the meaningful work it had taken her so long to find, or leave BPI and thereby turn her back perhaps forever on the possibility of a doctorate. Would she always be treated as a subordinate, beneath consideration, if she did not have a PhD?

She decided to risk it. She abandoned a doctorate two years into the process and committed herself entirely to the creation of new drugs, and soon the discoveries began flowing from her laboratory in an unreal procession that proved the merit of the new metabolic-based techniques that she and Hitchings had been developing. In 1950, she took a critical component of a compound used in the formation of DNA nucleotides and replaced one of its oxygen atoms with a sulfur atom, creating 6-mercaptopurine (6-MP). 6-MP is converted in the cell into thioinosine monophosphate (TIMP), which is itself just one atom different from inosine monophosphate (IMP), a critical gateway compound in the recycling and creation of adenine and guanine, two of the major components of DNA.

6-MP, then, introduces a non-functional compound, TIMP, in place of the necessary compound, IMP, and thereby throws a wrench in the cycle of DNA formation, which is precisely the sort of thing one would like to do for cells that are multiplying beyond all reason and require large amounts of DNA to do so, i.e., cancerous cells. In 1950, if you were a child and had leukaemia, there was more than a 60 per cent chance that you would be dead within a year. Yet 6-MP, given to child leukaemia patients, induced complete (though temporary) remission and on the strength of the preliminary data the drug was approved for release by 1953.

As it turned out, 6-MP by itself is insufficient to prevent relapse, as it needs to be combined in a cocktail with other drugs to target the cancer at several points, but in those combinations it is able not only to slow the progress of childhood leukaemia but to completely eradicate it in 80 per cent of cases.

Elion had found humanity's first drug that effectively combated one of our oldest foes, but she was not one to rest on her laurels. She continued to tinker with 6-MP and in 1957 created a variant, azathioprine, to deal with one of 6-MP's major shortcomings, the fact that it was broken down so quickly in the body. Azathioprine is not active until it is absorbed and slowly converted to 6-MP, thereby increasing the longevity of 6-MP within the relevant tissues. In 1958, a researcher named Robert Schwarz saw the potential of a purine-inhibiting drug like 6-MP to shut down the body's immune response against transplanted organs, and visited Elion to see if she had a more potent version of it. She gave him azathioprine and in clinical tests it proved precisely what was needed to prevent organ rejection. In 1962, it was used in conjunction with prednisone in the world's first successful kidney transplant operation, and was the central drug in organ transplants for the next two decades.

In 1967, Hitchings retired from Burroughs Wellcome and Elion had the chance to prove that her results were, in fact, the product of her own chemical insight. With characteristic daring, she decided to tackle a problem that the pharmaceutical industry had declared insoluble – developing an effective anti-viral medication. Two decades previously, in 1948, she had created a drug, aminopurine, before the discovery of 6-MP, that was effective against leukaemia but was so toxic it was not a feasible long-term treatment. It also had anti-viral characteristics, but at the time Elion was devoted to finding a leukaemia cure, and so let aminopurine lapse in obscurity until 1968, when she decided it might be a good starting point for developing the world's first anti-virus drug. Over the coming years, Elion and her research team followed the same methods that Elion and Hitchings had invented two decades before – find something that works, investigate the chemical pathways that it partakes in, and produce variant compounds that target crucial parts in those pathways and just those pathways.

The result of their research, revealed to the world after years of secrecy in 1974, was acyclovir. It is essentially inactive until a virus invades a cell. Then, viral enzymes change it into a form that inhibits viral DNA polymerase, preventing the virus from producing more viral DNA and thereby from making copies of itself, without interfering in any way with the cell's production of its own DNA. In effect, it tricks the virus into creating its own destroyer. It is cheap, non-toxic in most cases, and as of 2017 stands as the 166th most prescribed drug in the United States.

Elion retired in 1983, and in 1984 the team she had trained was responsible for the creation of AZT, the only drug available to treat AIDS until 1991. In 1988, she split the Nobel Prize in Physiology or Medicine with Hitchings and Sir James Black for their role in discovering new methods in the development of medications. Hitchings was none too thrilled to be sharing the award with somebody whom he considered to have been his subordinate, but the Nobel committee argued that her work after his departure in developing the world's first anti-viral drug was a *pretty good* sign that she was at least an equal actor in the work Burroughs Wellcome did in the 1950s and early 1960s. Elion continued to act in an advisory capacity to Burroughs Wellcome as well as teach classes in methodology at Duke University after her official retirement. Her last paper was published in 1998, one year before her sudden death (after collapsing while out on her daily walk).

There are numbers that sum up Elion's career – the forty-five patents, the over 231 scientific articles, the six decades of work, and there are numbers we can perhaps never calculate – the number of children cured of leukaemia, the number of lives saved due to a successful organ transplant, the number of people protected from opportunistic infections by an anti-viral drug, who owe their health to her dedication to investigating the fundamentals of biochemical interactions and her ability to see applications in new fields for variations of old compounds. She saw disease as a chain of chemical actions which could be tricked into self-termination by a sufficiently cunning series of cleverly disguised compounds, and spent her life getting the better of our most determined foes. Behind those drugs that save so many of us on a daily basis there was a determined and brilliant mind, and to that mind there belongs a face, one it is worth remembering, in times of sickness surely, but also in those of health.

Further Reading

There is not yet, for variously unfathomable reasons, a full-length non-juvenile treatment of Elion's life. Barring that, you can find a nice summary of her work in the as-ever indispensable *Nobel Prize Women in Science* by Sharon Bertsch McGrayne, and in various memorial articles written upon her death, such as the National Academy of Sciences biographical memoir by Mary Ellen Avery or the Royal Society biographical memoir published in Volume 54 in 2008.

Chapter 30

The Secret Life of Hormones

Rosalyn Yalow and the Discovery of Radioimmunoassaying

There is an unsung immensity in the craft of Measuring Things Better. Within our sparkling cleverness for developing better and better measurement tools there lies the secret of our advancement, not only as science-doers but as a species generally. The dramatic potential for improving human life through better measurement has few grander success stories than that of Rosalyn Yalow (1921–2011), co-discoverer of Radioimmunoassaying (RIA), the technique that not only solved the mystery of what Type II Diabetes is all about, but also more or less invented the field of modern endocrinology.

Throughout the 1950s, Yalow worked with the several shades too brilliant Solomon Berson in developing new methods to measure first the flow of blood, and then the flow of substances within the blood, using newly available radioactive isotopes as markers. It was a novel approach to a problem that had been previously studied by cutting major arteries of condemned criminals, and catching the blood in a graduated bucket. Knife, Stopwatch, Science.

The Bucket Method was not terribly accurate and, sad to say, it was not an isolated case of the American medical establishment using criminals for non-consensual testing prior to, and even well after, the Second World War. The work that Yalow did on blood flow and on the products of the thyroid gland (which also did not take heed of the notion of Medical Consent, we should note, though she did everything she could to minimise the danger to the subject) gave her, a nuclear physicist by education, the practical training in preparing and measuring radioactive isotopes for what would become the great discovery of her life.

For there was a terrible mystery at the time surrounding Type II Diabetes. Whereas Type I was relatively well understood as resulting from an insufficiency of insulin in the blood, and could therefore be treated by regular injection of pig insulin, Type II was a bit baffling. Those suffering seemed to be producing insulin just fine, and yet still had the same issues with blood sugar maintenance as those suffering from Type I. To get to the bottom of the mystery, somebody had to find a way to measure the amount of insulin in the blood at different times.

This was, to put it mildly, difficult. Insulin exists in miniscule quantities in the blood, far too dilute for any technique of the time to detect. So, Yalow and Berson developed a deliciously simple hack that formed the basis for an entire industry or twelve. They discovered that, when they injected insulin that had been radioactively tagged into the body of a person who had been receiving insulin injections, those tagged insulin molecules were latched on to by globulin molecules, which they soon realised were antibodies produced by the host.

That was controversial enough. Insulin is, relatively speaking, a small molecule, and the medical wisdom of the day said that only massive molecules could trigger antibody responses. In their landmark paper of 1956, Yalow and Berson even had to remove the word 'antibody' from their prospective title in order to publish the article. But while the scientific community was huffing about their radical results, Yalow and Berson pushed on with a critical insight.

They saw that a patient's native insulin, when present, also occupied space on these antibodies and therefore knew that, if you took a sample of patient blood, and mixed it with antibodies and radioactively tagged insulin, you could tell how much insulin was in the blood by measuring the ratio of radioactive insulin molecules wrapped up by an antibody to those left alone in solution. The more radioactive isotope in solution, the more native insulin there must be.

So, as long as any substance has a corresponding binding molecule, be it an antibody or something similar (as in the case with the B12 assaying later done in the Yalow-Berson laboratory), you can use RIA to measure the concentration of that substance by producing a radioactive copy, and setting it into competition with its natural counterpart for space on the binding molecule. As the common metaphor runs, it is hormonal musical chairs. Measure the radioactive kids left standing on their own, chairless, and you have at last a measure of how many 'normal' kids there must be, seated but invisible.

Yalow and Berson refused to patent their methods, believing them too important to the future of medicine to be owned by anybody. And so, people around the world flew to reproduce the success of Yalow's insulin experiments with other hitherto unmeasurable hormones and peptides. The great blank book of the endocrine system unfolded itself under RIA methods, and after Berson died, Yalow deepened the search to the brain, finding peptides that served as neurotransmitters, and therefore giving us a whole new perspective on the major players of neurochemistry. By finding a new way of measuring incredibly dilute and relatively lightweight solutes, Yalow gifted humanity all of the improvements in the treatment of disease that have come from the expansion of our hormonal and neurochemical arsenal.

All well and good, but where is the brisk summary of her life, the anecdotes of her growing years, the personal moments of emotional depth?

They are not here, and will not be. Rosalyn Yalow, unique among the scientists we have looked at so far, IS her work. A headstrong daughter of Depression-era Jewish immigrant stock dubbed The Queen Bee by her family, she knew exactly what she wanted from an early age – a life devoted to science, and a family who recognised the primacy that science had in her life and did not question her decisions.

Through unadulterated force of will, she attained both. Her husband, Aaron Yalow, a physicist himself and ultra-Orthodox Jew, worshipped her and made a deal with her that, as long as she kept a kosher household, he would give her free rein in all other areas of life. Her children understood that, in matters of sentiment or humour or vulnerability, they were to look to their father, as their mother simply did not have those qualities and did not care to have them. She did not form deep relationships with other women, had no side interests or hobbies, never told jokes, and spent every available moment in her laboratory with Sol Berson. She was on a mission to show that a woman could have a family and still do top-quality research, and in her need to appear perfect, had a tendency to discount the troubles of those close to her. The roll call of her life features a steady stream of awards and honours after her and Berson's landmark 1956 paper, culminating in the 1977 Nobel Prize, and an impressive array of discoveries well into her sixties, but few moments of purely personal connection with other humans.

One would like to think that this was simply her way, that she did not feel the lack of human warmth because she was not interested in it, that her mind and heart were completely satisfied by her work and her reputation as a perfect human who raised an immaculate family with one hand while solving the world's endocrinology problems with the other. The darker possibility, that she felt the loss but tucked it deep away, knowing that any sign of weakness would hurt the chances of later women pursuing a career in medicine, that she sacrificed herself tirelessly for the greater cause of expanding opportunity, is perhaps testified to by the deep but quickly sublimated loss she felt upon the early death of Berson in 1972, and her lifelong drive to make sure that his name was mentioned with hers any time their work in RIA was mentioned.

Yalow officially retired at age 70, in 1991, but continued keeping an office at the Bronx VA even after the effects of strokes and a broken hip had rendered her all but immobile, accepting invitations to speak about the future of women in science, the importance of nuclear research, and the need for more public medical funding. Her work was done in that grand spirit of public medicine that was swallowed whole with the development of pharmaceutical monopolies in the 1960s and 1970s, a time when young researchers still had options outside of industry for making a steady and honourable living, a time that Yalow brought alluringly to life each time she spoke of the glory days, working on a shoestring budget in a makeshift laboratory with Solomon Berson to understand the hidden world of hormone regulation.

Rosalyn Sussman Yalow died in 2011 in The Bronx.

Further Reading

Eugene Straus's *Rosalyn Yalow: Nobel Laureate. Her Life and Work in Medicine* is a great source from somebody who worked closely with her for a long period, and observed astutely her relationship with her children and colleagues. It treats us to long personal reflections from both of her children, and a deeply sad account of how, at the age of 75, she was dumped at a hospital after a severe stroke. The chronology hops around a bit, which is narratively interesting but makes it a bit difficult to nail down the relative sequence of events in her life, but the scientific explanations are clearly and elegantly stated.

Chapter 31

Ancient Secrets, Modern Methods

Nobel Laureate Tu Youyou, Malaria, and the Discovery of Artemisinin

In 1955, the World Health Organization had what, on the surface, seemed a splendid idea: Let's Get Rid of Malaria. Just four years earlier, the United States, after a concentrated anti-malarial programming that involved the spraying of 4.5 *million* houses with 1939's Miracle Insecticide DDT, had declared malaria definitively eradicated – why not use similar methods on a global scale to defeat the disease once and for all?

Why not indeed.

The WHO gave it their best shot, coordinating, with varying degrees of success, efforts to spray malaria-carrying mosquitoes into extinction alongside more everyday mosquito abatement programmes. It went well at first, but the uneven application of the methods, the migrations caused by war, and the existence of countries which refused treatment altogether resulted in something fearful: the rise of a strain of malaria parasite, *plasmodium falciparum*, which was entirely resistant to the quinine medications that were humanity's only real effective defence against the disease.

The impact was not long in making itself felt: in the jungles of south-east Asia, where American and Vietnamese troops slogged through mosquito-ridden jungles, the number of malaria cases began a precipitous climb. The Americans lunged forward in a mad search for a cure that combed through over 200,000 potential drugs, with no luck, while in China a woman who combined the rigour of Western pharmacological training with an awareness of the traditions of Chinese medicine discovered after many trials and many more tribulations the plant that could stand up to the parasite.

Tu Youyou's (b. 1930) life spans China's greatest convulsions and acts of tragic self-definition. Born in the brief respite between Chiang Kai-Shek's consolidation of North and Central China in 1927 and the invasion by the Japanese in 1937, Tu as the only girl in a family of boys might have expected domesticity as her lot in life, but in fact was sent to a series of private schools by her parents to get the very best education available. Speaking of this time in her Nobel memoirs, she mentions every school she attended, but curiously, and perhaps portentously, makes no mention of the impact on her life of the 1937 invasion by the Japanese of her home town.

Besides the technical details of her schooling, we know little of Tu's early years until she contracted tuberculosis at the age of 16. It knocked her out of school for two years and gave her a compass with which to steer her life: she would devote herself to the study of medicine. Recovering at last in 1948, she made up for lost time, finished high school by 1951, and was on her way to Peking University to major in pharmacognosy – the study of medicinal drugs derived from natural sources such as plants. Here she picked up crucial training in how different plants responded to different extraction techniques that would form a central part of her great discovery two decades later. She also learned, from a Western perspective, how drugs operate on the body, which gave her new insights into the world and the assumptions of traditional Chinese medicine.

In 1955, the Chinese Ministry of Health opened up a new academy, the Academy of Traditional Chinese Medicine (ATCM), and it was here that Tu found her first work directly out of university, and where she would do the work that saved millions of lives and made herself the first Chinese woman ever to win a Nobel Prize. In an effort to improve the state of medicine in China, the government heavily encouraged cross-communication between Western-educated doctors and practitioners of traditional Chinese medicine, each contributing their best insights to foster the development and improvement of the other.

After spending her first professional years analysing the properties of traditional cures for flatworms, Tu was sent on a three-year intensive course in traditional Chinese medicine in 1959, emerging at precisely the point when the need for new anti-malarial drugs was most profoundly felt. In 1964, Ho Chi Minh asked Mao Zedong to devote resources to the finding of a new cure for malaria, resulting in 1967 in the secret creation of Project 523. It was the red-hot beginning of the Cultural Revolution, a time when scientists were suspected of being fundamentally bourgeois and anti-Communist. In the decade that followed, over a million accused 'bourgeois sympathisers' died while as many as 10 million more academics, researchers and members of the intelligentsia were assigned to manual labour in remote parts of the country.

Tu, at the age of just 39, was given charge of the ATCM's effort to find an anti-malarial drug, a position of great visibility and importance with corresponding pressures to perform. Her husband had been sent away to the countryside as part of the governmental programme to compel urbanites to develop rural skills, and she had to give her 4-year-old daughter to her parents, and place her 1-year-old daughter in the custody of a family who ran a daycare centre, in order to attend to her new work. When she finally got to visit her older daughter three years later, the child did not recognise her.

But there was plenty of work to fill the void – Tu compiled a list of 2,000 possible malaria remedies culled from the last couple of millennia of Chinese medical writings, and her team set to work to prepare and test the most promising. *Artemisia annua*, or sweet wormwood, was found all over the historical records and yet in testing the only thing consistent was the inconsistency of its efficacy. It was in danger of being abandoned altogether when Tu had her crucial insight: combining her knowledge of extraction methods with her close reading of the original texts with her insight into variables that can impact drug potency, she came to the conclusion that the extraction process for *Artemisia annua* was fundamentally flawed. Traditionally, plants were boiled in water to extract the compounds that had medicinal properties, but Tu believed the high temperature was adversely affecting the ability of the compound to function, and opted for a method using ethyl ether which required a much lower temperature.

The change in method made all the difference. In animal trials, the new drug showed a 100 per cent efficacy and, in order to overcome doubts about its impact on the human respiratory and circulatory systems, Tu volunteered to be the first human to take the drug. Working around the clock in close quarters that adversely affected the health of her team, samples of the drug we now know as artemisinin were prepared for test trials while Tu carried out the analysis to discover its chemical nature.

In the process of those analytical studies, she managed to synthesise a second drug, dihydroartemisinin, almost entirely by accident in 1973, and in trials she discovered it was ten times more effective against malaria than artemisinin. After almost interminable rounds of interdepartmental meetings, administrative flowchart adjustments, and trial review, the existence and structure of artemisinin were formally announced in 1979, a decade after Tu first was charged with finding a new cure for malaria.

The discovery of artemisinin was a major breakthrough that saved millions of lives, but its discoverer languished in almost perfect obscurity until she won the Lasker Prize in 2011 and the Nobel Prize in 2015, becoming the first Chinese scientist to win a Nobel in Medicine, and the first woman in China to win a Nobel in any field. For a hint as to why the years 1979 to 2011 represent such a void in the historical record, we can look to *Tu*

Youyou and the Discovery of Artemisinin (2017) by Yi Rao, Daqing Zhang and Runhong Li. The book purports to be primarily about Tu, but in fact she is scarcely present in its pages, the majority being given over to minute descriptions of committee structures and an overarching emphasis on the bureaucratic flow of communication that dominated Project 523. This focus on the bureaucracy of Chinese science in the 1960s and 1970s at the expense of the individuals within is both fascinating to behold and characteristic of a philosophy of the heroism of collective effort, but also results inevitably in the diminution of any relevant individuals like Tu.

Her youth had been spent in times of war and revolution, sometimes in sickness but always in study. Her most productive years saw her separated from her family so that she could carry on work that ultimately saved millions of lives. Her autumn brought her official honours in China and creeping obscurity in the rest of the world until finally, at the age of 85, she was vaulted into prominence as an example of what Chinese medical science could accomplish when properly directed. Through her, two massive traditions looked at each other for a moment and found common cause, and eventual triumph. As she heads to her ninetieth year, Tu continues to advocate for stretching that moment into an era, one of discovery and understanding as history and modernity trade their insights and push their shared world forward.

Further Reading

The book by Yi, Daqing and Runhong mentioned above is, as I said, fascinating as a glimpse into the bureaucratic focus on Chinese medical research in the midst of the Cultural Revolution, but is absolute rubbish as a book about Tu Youyou. There is nothing about her life before artemisinin, nothing about it after, and the time in between the mixture is about 97 per cent mind-numbingly dull flow charts about administrative reporting responsibilities between government agencies and 3 per cent repetitions of the same couple of research facts about Tu's process. As a biography of a woman scientist, it is probably the worst I have ever read. So save your money and check out her Nobel memoir, which you can find on the Nobel Prize's website.

Chapter 32

One Doctor Against Nuclear War

Helen Caldicott and the Creation of the Physicians for Social Responsibility

It might be difficult to believe if you were born within the last three decades, but there was once a time when America was led by a doddering former B-List celebrity who clung to popularity via an intoxicating and ever-fluctuating combination of charisma and fear-mongering, culminating in a mad push for producing stockpiles of nuclear weapons that could kill every person on Earth multiple times over, should the occasion arise. The Soviet Union and the United States had been locked in a half-century tournament of mutual and wilful misunderstanding perpetuated by a succession of leaders who took it as gospel that a nuclear war was winnable, so long as you were the guy with the most weapons.

Fortunately, we learned our lesson from the dangerous seduction of Cold War thinking, and would *certainly* never fall for that trick again, but it was a rare person indeed in the 1970s and early 1980s who could see beyond the rhetoric of the Strategic Air Command's 'Our Profession is Peace' sloganeering and soberly calculate the cost to humanity if we should fail to rise above our worst demons. There were early detractors of nuclear warfare, surely, but they were easily sloughed off as Commie poets – layabout peaceniks too treacherous or uninformed to see the Real Danger of the Soviet Union and the Real Security to be had behind a wall of atomic weaponry.

If the dangers of nuclear war were to be discussed openly, it would have to be by a segment of the population people trusted, people who had something to lose by their anti-nuclear advocacy and thus could only be speaking out of dire earnest for the public good. In 1978, the medical community assumed responsibility for that role when Dr Helen Caldicott (b. 1938), an Australian physician and cystic fibrosis specialist who had spent the last half decade studying the medical impact of radiation and nuclear weaponry, formed the Physicians for Social Responsibility (PSR), an organisation of medical men and women who would form the anti-nuclear intellectual vanguard in the closing years of the Cold War.

Forty years before the founding of the PSR, Helen Caldicott had been born Helen Broinowski, the first of three children. The Broinowskis were an intellectually adventurous, quick-tempered couple, and Helen's mother in particular alternated between long stretches of reading and short bursts of rage directed at her eldest daughter. Helen was regularly beaten throughout childhood, and as is often the case with maltreated children, she carried with her a constant sense of guilt: if Mother is treating me this badly this often surely I must be to blame?

Physically and emotionally battered, young Helen was nonetheless given free rein to expand her mind academically and intellectually. When she announced at a young age her intention of becoming a doctor, she was encouraged by both parents and sent to an expensive preparatory academy, in spite of the slim financial situation of the family. The Australian educational system at the time allowed one to attend medical school directly after high school, and so in 1961, at the mere age of 23, she emerged from the University of Adelaide with a medical degree.

The landmark event in Caldicott's life that year was not her graduation, however, but the death of her father after a sharp and sudden downturn in his health. It was a devastating loss of a parent, ally and kindred spirit, and, in her despair, she turned perhaps too ready an ear to the wooing of a young radiologist named William Caldicott. Unlike the pattern in her previous relationships, she was not madly in love with him, but he was sociable and amusing, was of her own profession and in short, he made the loneliness of loss less oppressive. They were married within a year of her father's death.

The newlyweds proceeded to have three children in quick succession, and Caldicott had to manage cooking, childcare and profession at once, a task which reached its crescendo of difficulty when William took a tempting position in Boston while she was still pregnant, forcing her to look after the children, have a new child, and manage the move of all the children to rejoin him in America, with nobody to rely on except her seriously ailing mother.

Somehow, she fought through that episode and made it to the United States with children and mother in tow. For five years, she tried various configurations of family, work and political engagement, each more exhausting and demanding than the last. She witnessed America's success in increasing the life expectancy for patients with cystic fibrosis, and wanted to import those methods to Australia, where a They're Doomed, The Best

Thing Is To Let Them Die Quickly strategy was in place that brought with it a life expectancy dramatically less than equivalent patients in the United States.

This work was important, and the cystic fibrosis clinic she eventually established became a model for what might be done to improve the lives of Australian CF patients and their families, but the cause that consumed the rest of Caldicott's life arrived at last in 1971 in the form of a mushroom cloud. The French were performing nuclear tests in the Pacific that were causing radioactive fallout to pepper mainland Australia. Caldicott read up on the health risks not only directly caused by the detonation of the weapons but inflicted on those who mine the uranium required for them, and the communities who live in the vicinity of those mines.

With every moment that could be spared from her medical practice, she was out on the road speaking to whoever would listen about the medical effects of radioactive fallout and even casual, regular exposure to radioactive materials. When the family returned to America for a sabbatical year in 1975, she set herself the task of confronting the most powerfully held belief of the world's most powerful nation: that the nuclear bomb was the United States' best and only chance at security and peace.

She earned a reputation as a speaker who could tailor an impromptu speech to the cut of her audience on the fly – now cool, professional and statistical when speaking before a collection of medical professionals, then passionate and maternal addressing a mother's organisation, and later full of Gospel truths about peace and forgiveness when holding the attention of the nation's manifold religious gatherings.

As she drew larger crowds at higher profile venues, Caldicott realised that her position as a physician gave her words a weight unavailable to most of the anti-nuclear movement. Those willing to write off poets and social theorists and environmentalists as anti-American Communist sympathisers suddenly found themselves open to the words of a medical person explaining the medical issues attendant upon the development and use of nuclear weapons. The next step seemed clear – to band together as many medical professionals as possible in an organisation that might present a united front against nuclear weapons. The first meeting of this organisation, the Physicians for Social Responsibility, which would at its height claim tens of thousands of members, was held in the Caldicott home and consisted of less than half a dozen attendees.

For five years, Caldicott criss-crossed the United States, taking every invitation to appear on television and before concerned citizens to present the human cost of nuclear proliferation. After the Three Mile nuclear incident of 1979, she realised she could not balance her work as a physician with her role as leader of the nascent anti-nuclear movement, and decided that the latter was where she needed to be. She became a full-time anti-nuclear advocate, appearing regularly on all the major networks, sometimes flanked by famous anti-nuclear celebrities like Sally Field or Lily Tomlin.

After one talk, she was approached by the daughter of President Ronald Reagan, begging her to please talk with her father about the dangers of his administration's nuclear policy. The resulting one-on-one talk with the president was among the most surreal moments of Caldicott's life as Reagan blurred in and out of focus, mixing up his numbers and sources but adamantly maintaining his administration's policy. It was a depressing meeting, and worse was to come for Caldicott and the anti-nuclear movement.

As the PSR grew in membership and influence, various high-placed individuals within its ranks began forming plans to seize power from Caldicott, first by forming a splinter organisation, the International Physicians for the Prevention of Nuclear War (IPPNW), which directly competed with PSR for funding and deliberately locked Caldicott out from its power structure, and then by fomenting dissatisfaction within the PSR at Caldicott's style of leadership. She had shouldered most of the burden for publicising the PSR's position in the media and for travelling the country drumming up new membership, primarily because nobody else stepped forward to do that kind of boots on the ground work, but now she faced criticism for being too often in front of the cameras, and for the emotionality of some of her appeals. In 1983, the Board of Directors said it would be better for her to leave the presidency, which she duly did.

Luckily, another organisation she had founded in 1980, Women's Action for Nuclear Disarmament (WAND), was more than happy to have a greater share of her time, and together they lobbied hard for the election of Walter Mondale in 1984, only to stand by in disbelief as he refused to offer a definitive policy of nuclear disarmament that might have energised his voter base. His monumental defeat put the movement in temporary paralysis, and Caldicott with it. For the first time, she faced complete doubt about the utility of everything she had ever done. While the IPPNW spent its energy lobbying for a Nobel Prize for itself (which it won), Caldicott lamented that, in spite of the PSR, WAND and the IPPNW, in spite of their massive public demonstrations and tens of thousands of members, not a single nuclear weapon had been decommissioned as a result of their half decade of work.

It was a low point, and it would get lower. Her husband William was doing medical work he found unstimulating, and was growing lonely and resentful as Caldicott took every opportunity to speak publicly about the anti-nuclear movement, leaving him as the primary caretaker of the children. They sought counselling, but to no avail. He left her in 1988.

All was not, however, for naught. The organisations she had raised to prominence from nothing had not directly pushed through a policy to denuclearise the world in their first half decade of existence, but their message had broken through the nuclear mania of the Cold War, and by the mid-1980s polling data showed overwhelming support for a freeze on the production of nuclear weapons, and a policy of steady nuclear disarmament, a shift so dramatic that Reagan's handlers initiated a paradigm shift in nuclear policy that combined with Mikhail Gorbachev's earnest hatred of nuclear weapons to produce some first steps towards meaningful nuclear change.

Yes, Caldicott was no longer president of the PSR, but that also meant she was no longer beholden to the restrictions they wanted to place on her message, and when she re-emerged as a speaker on nuclear issues, her themes took on a broader scope. She challenged assumptions about the safety of nuclear power which she had been repeatedly dissuaded from tackling in the heyday of the PSR, and developed themes about America's irresponsible hunger for energy that keep us dependent on large-scale energy resources.

The Cold War is over, but Dr Helen Caldicott is decidedly still here, and will continue to be so long as nations take their capacity to destroy as the measure of their strength, and the prospective elimination of Other People as the guarantor of their safety.

Further Reading

Caldicott has written a number of books, each responding to that era's nuclear policy. The first, *Nuclear Madness* (1978), is still her most famous, while Caldicott's post-PSR freedom allowed her to evolve her position, resulting in *Nuclear Power is Not the Answer* (2006) and a small fleet of other titles besides. For the meteoric path of her life, her autobiography *Desperate Passion* (1996) is a brutally frank and self-analytic portrait of the birth of the anti-nuclear movement and her own trials of depression attempting to incorporate activism, childhood trauma, parental death, career, family and marriage into something like a stable life. There were also several films made about her at the height of the PSR, *Eight Minutes to Midnight* (1981) and *If You Love This Planet* (1982) being the two easiest to find. There are also plenty of full speeches from throughout her career, available on YouTube.

Chapter 33

Françoise Barré-Sinoussi, the Discovery of HIV, and the Fight Against AIDS

Pandemics. Having raised their heads every century or so to spread primal panic and horror on a continental scale, they were something we believed ourselves well rid of by the mid-twentieth century. By vaccine and vitamin, sanitation and antibiotic, humans had pushed back the terrors of globe-spanning disease in the first world and had every reason to expect that, if a new bug should dare raise its head, it would be summarily identified and executed before it had a chance to penetrate Main Street. Then, on 5 June 1981, we had the first inkling of how wrong, how very wrong, we were.

On that day, the Center for Disease Control announced five cases of severe immunodeficiency in Los Angeles, a number that grew to 270 by year's end. Previously healthy individuals were being felled by advantageous diseases that their immune systems should have had no trouble dispatching. These cases of catastrophic immune system failure, at first seemingly limited to homosexuals and heroin users, soon spread into all communities the world over, as 270 cases became 20,000 by the end of 1985, became 300,000 by 1990, and today stands at 70 million infected individuals across the world.

As the first disease reports trickled through the medical community, there was a grim and general realisation that not only did we not know how to combat this disease – we did not even know what it was. One man, however, had a hunch. His name was Willy Rozenbaum and he believed the symptoms of this new disease matched up with one discovered in 1980 by Gallo, Hinuma and Yoshida: Human T Lymphotropic Virus (HTLV). In 1982, he went to the Pasteur Institute to find somebody experienced enough in retrovirus analysis to test his theory. He was soon passed along to the laboratory of Jean-Claude Chermann, where a tiny group of researchers was studying the role retroviruses play in certain forms of leukaemia, a group that included the woman destined to discover the culprit behind AIDS and to dedicate the next decades of her life to coordinating the world's resources to eradicating it: Françoise Barré-Sinoussi.

Born in Paris in 1947, her family was of Parisian extraction stretching back generations, but her most prized memories were of vacation trips to the countryside where she could wander and observe plants and animals by herself, or compete in pet snail races with her cousin (whenever her snail lost, she felt it must, of course, be due to a terrible snail illness, and set herself the task of diagnosing the malady). She knew that she wanted to do something with the 'living' sciences, but could not decide between pure biology and medicine. Reasoning that a degree in biology would take less time and therefore be cheaper for her parents, she ultimately decided on biology, her head full of dreams of stimulating laboratory work.

Imagine her disappointment, then, when her first years were focused almost entirely on theory, with virtually no laboratory work at all. After two years, she was ready to leave the university and join a laboratory tech training college just to finally have practical research work to do, when fate intervened in the form of the college president. He told her that, having already finished two years at the university, it was inadvisable to stop now to join his school's programme. For her own good, he turned her down, and so it was back to the university, and theory.

But Barré-Sinoussi was not one to accept defeat so easily. She spread a wide net, looking for laboratories who would take her while she continued her university studies, and in 1970 she found a spot in the small but well-regarded laboratory of Jean-Claude Chermann, a virologist working on retroviruses that caused leukaemia in mice. In spite of her lack of laboratory experience, Chermann took her into his laboratory family and acted as her mentor. She spent as little time as possible actually in class in order to spend more at Chermann's laboratory and learn all the tools and tricks of a retrovirologist.

All of which begs the question, what is a retrovirus? Remember that there are two main carriers of genetic information: DNA and RNA. Most living things keep a permanent copy of their genetic structure in the form of double-stranded DNA and use single-stranded RNA for various tasks in the creation of proteins and regulation of the cell.

Retroviruses, however, carry RNA, not DNA, as their primary genetic source. When they invade a cell, they make DNA copies of their RNA and insert those copies into the host DNA. The host cell then believes the foreign DNA is part of its own code, and happily copies it over and over again, creating new copies of everything needed to make a swarm of new retroviruses, which will invade new healthy cells, thereby triggering a biological chain reaction. As infectious agents, retroviruses are particularly nasty as the process that produces viral genetic copies is notoriously imprecise, generating progeny viruses with mutational variations that immune systems have difficulty keeping up with.

Barré-Sinoussi received her PhD in 1975 and continued at the Pasteur Institute, researching retroviruses until the fateful day when Rozenbaum's challenge made its way to her desk. A momentous decision had to be made: would she work on the assumption that the disease agent was HTLV, and proceed through the established steps laid out for its identification, or would she start from step one and push her way through the various methods and tactics for identifying a new infective agent? Not entirely convinced by Rozenbaum's claim, she opted for the latter, securing on his advice some samples from a patient exhibiting symptoms of swollen lymph nodes that often marked the onset of the new disease.

Analysing the samples, she noted the presence of reverse transcriptase which betokens retroviral activity, but simultaneously noticed that the T-Cells she was studying were dying out at an alarming rate, too fast to gather the corroborating data she needed. The laboratory team put their heads together and had a brilliant flash of insight – why not go over to the local blood bank and ask them for fresh blood? There would be enough white cells there for the virus to hopefully feed on, which would extend the amount of time they could study the original viral sample.

The trick worked. Retrovirus activity picked up, and new knowledge was gained: whatever this disease was, it clearly had the ability to infect and eventually destroy new white blood cells. Barré-Sinoussi was convinced that what she had was a retrovirus, but was it HTLV? She got in contact with Robert Gallo, one of the original discoverers of HTLV, and asked him for his help. Obligingly, he sent her samples of the HTLV retrovirus and of antibodies that responded to its presence. Using these samples, she discovered that the HTLV antibodies did not interact with her retrovirus, and the antibodies from the original patient did not respond to HTLV. Whatever this new disease was, it was not caused by HTLV.

All this research was carried out at breakneck speed. Rozenbaum had laid out his idea in December 1982. Barré-Sinoussi started testing in January 1983, and her paper identifying HIV was published in May of that year, a startling turn-around built on the cleverness of her colleagues, and the inspired solidity of her retroviral analytic technique. She would go on to win the Nobel Prize in 2008 for the discovery, but in the meantime, there was work to be done.

Africa, where AIDS probably originated, had by and large kept quiet about the epidemic in its midst. Fearful for the political and economic ramifications if the disease were known and its scale laid out, pressure was put on local health services to remain silent about immunodeficiency-related deaths. Part of the task Barré-Sinoussi set for herself, then, was to determine the scope of the African AIDS epidemic and coordinate resources to allow large-scale testing and treatment to be carried out throughout the continent. She travelled across Africa, and eventually south-east Asia as well, assessing the tremendous need for better public education about the causes and transmission of AIDS, and establishing centres that could identify AIDS cases early and administer life-saving anti-retroviral treatments.

It was work of profound importance and substantial frustration. For every government like Thailand or Brazil that worked vigorously with her teams to educate the public and catch early cases before they became fatal, there were governments like Thabo Mbeki's South Africa which, seizing upon the HIV denialist theories of UC Berkeley biologist Peter Duesberg, declared that AIDS was caused by issues of sanitation, malnutrition and lifestyle, not by the HIV virus. As a result, the government refused to institute early detection or anti-retroviral programmes, ultimately causing hundreds of thousands to die unnecessarily.

Somehow amidst travelling the world in an unflagging attempt to create a stable international approach to AIDS treatment, Barré-Sinoussi's research carries on, investigating the genetic variations that allow some members of the population to seemingly purge HIV from their system naturally. Unlike normal people infected by HIV, who must take anti-retroviral medication for their entire lives, these 'elite controllers', who make up less than 0.3 per cent of the population, are able to safely stop taking their medication and not experience a relapse of AIDS symptoms. Learning from their biological bag of tricks could hold the key for single-trial medications and perhaps even the long-sought AIDS vaccine.

In the meantime, Barré-Sinoussi can point with satisfaction to the sharp increase in anti-retroviral treatment resulting in no small part from her efforts in working with foreign governments to create public health policies based on good science but still responsive to local concerns and methods. In 2002, fewer than 400,000 people in developing countries were receiving anti-retroviral treatment. Ten years later, thanks to Barré-Sinoussi and others like her, that number had grown to 6.5 million individuals. In Africa, without treatment, 40 per cent of infected mothers passed HIV directly to their babies, a number that now stands at less than 5 per cent.

There are people who have done so much good, who have so unambiguously made the world a better place by the work of their mind and heart, that finding the words to sum their lives is an impossible task. If Françoise Barré-Sinoussi were *just* the researcher who discovered HIV and is looking into genetic causes of HIV resistance, or *just* the voyager who went into the heart of the countries most impacted by AIDS to evaluate what needed to be done to stop the omnipresent suffering, or *just* the organiser assembling experts from the world over to concentrate financial and intellectual resources in the fight against AIDS, or even *just* the spokesperson who uses her platform to educate the first and third worlds about what is being done, and what yet remains to be done, it would be enough to earn thanks. But she is all of those people at once, and before that, dumbstruck awe is all one can reasonably feel. Words are too small to express the thanks we owe, too small by half.

Further Reading

Francois Barré-Sinoussi's memoir/report on the history and future of AIDS treatment, *Pour un Monde Sans SIDA: Un Combat Partagé* (2012) is delightful and inspiring. It is all done in an interview format and I would say about a third of the book is devoted to her life and work, and the other two-thirds to investigating the world AIDS situation, and promising lines of research in new treatments and potential cures. It is in French, but the vocabulary is nowhere so technical as to be opaque, so a casual French reader should not have too much trouble with it.

Chapter 34

An ER Doctor in Space

The Story of Astronaut Rhea Seddon

The first astronaut class to include women candidates, announced in 1978 and self-dubbed the TFNG, or Thirty-Five New Guys, brought six women into the variously welcome glare of public scrutiny. Each of those six was a remarkable individual, but over time we have privileged in our memory those of them whose name is attached to some national or human first.

We remember Sally Ride, the first American woman in space, and Kathryn Sullivan, the first American woman to perform a spacewalk.

We remember Anna Fisher, the first mother in space, Shannon Lucid, the first woman to undertake a long-duration spaceflight, and Judith Resnik, both because she was the first Jewish American in space, and because of her tragic end aboard the space shuttle *Challenger*.

But what of that sixth astronaut, Dr Rhea Seddon? Lacking asterisk or acronym (though admittedly Sally Ride's FAWIS (First American Woman in Space) does not precisely flow off the tongue), need we relegate her to the faceless ranks of the Alsos, those who were not first at a thing and therefore deserve all of the inattention our worn and tired brains can muster?

We need not, and it would be a true shame were we to do so, because Seddon's story is an incredible one. At one point in her career, she was simultaneously an ER doctor, an astronaut, an astronaut's spouse (a job in and of itself with unique unpaid duties and responsibilities), and a mother. She went into space three times, two of them on Spacelab missions, was the first woman to hold the position of Technical Assistant to the Director (popularly called The Bubba), served on the Astronaut Selection Board, and worked as both CAPCOM (Capsule Communicator) and payload commander.

For somebody who served in so many different capacities during NASA's space shuttle era, her early story contains little that would hint of the stars as her ultimate life's destination. Born in 1947 in Murfreesboro, Tennessee, she was the inheritor of a tradition of Southern gentility that was rapidly being superseded by the educational demands and opportunities of the Space Age. She went to a Catholic elementary school, where an outside teacher was engaged to give the children the instruction they needed to be competitive in this new world that stressed technological competence over classical refinements and impeccable manners.

Science, it turned out, was something that came naturally to Seddon, and by the time she attended Murfreesboro High School she had decided that, if it were at all possible for a woman to do so in 1960s America, she would like to make science her vocation, and after a summer working in the office of Dr Lois Kennedy, she saw the life sciences in particular as her probable specialty. On the advice of a family friend, she decided to apply to Californian universities, and in 1965 arrived at UC Berkeley, a refined Southerner, devoted Christian, former cheerleader, science enthusiast and all-round workaholic who was about to touch down directly in the epicentre of the student protest movement of the late 1960s.

It must have been a cultural adjustment, to say the least, but in her memoirs, Seddon relates that she pushed through the turmoil, tear gas and omnipresent newness by putting her head down and ploughing forward with the work at hand. Totally alone and fending for herself in one of the nation's most prestigious pre-med programmes, she pushed through her difficulties and self-doubt and found herself working during a summer for the surgical suite at Rutherford County Hospital, where she discovered a deep interest in and fascination for surgery.

After receiving her physiology degree from Berkeley in 1970, she attended the University of Tennessee College of Medicine, one of six women in a class of a hundred. Thence began the usual horrors of an early medical career, the internships, residencies and moonlighting that collectively result in 100-hour working weeks experienced as blurs of intense life-or-death decisions alternating with the steady press of paperwork and the insistent thought, picking at the worn defences of a frazzled mind, 'Is this what you want your life to be?'

For most of us, psychological survival is predicated on vigorously suppressing that question, because for most of us nothing good could come of it. Either you are living the life you want (fun fact: you are not), or you are not but it is far too late to change and all that has been gained by asking the question is to make you feel miserable about something you are stuck with. Usually, then, humans are good at deflecting that thought, but one day, in the middle of an interminable shift, while sitting in the bare bones doctor's lounge, a co-worker asked Seddon what she would like to do, if she could do anything with her life, and from seemingly nowhere she replied, An Astronaut. As it happened, that co-worker once worked for NASA himself, and when, in 1977, NASA announced it was looking for the first new crop of astronauts in just under a decade, he noticed and passed the announcement on to Seddon.

This new group was not going to be composed exclusively of test pilots cut from essentially the same military cloth, but it would feature Mission Specialists, whose job was to run various experiments and technical tasks on the space shuttle, a new, reusable space vehicle that would balance original scientific research with paying satellite deployment missions for private industry and the military. These specialists need not be pilots or at the height of possible human fitness, but instead could be simply scientists of good reputation and reasonable fitness working in interesting fields that might tangentially be related to the conquest of space. Though she strongly doubted she would be admitted, Seddon submitted her application and carried on with her life.

Against her own expectations, however, she was selected, and the ER physician from Tennessee joined biochemist Shannon Lucid, engineer Judy Resnik, physician Anna Fisher, astrophysicist Sally Ride, and geologist Kathryn Sullivan in the class of the Thirty-Five New Guys revealed to the world in January 1978. Another member of that class was former Vietnam combat pilot Hoot Gibson, whom Seddon would go on to marry, making Gibson and Seddon the nation's first married astronaut couple, and effectively doubling each of their workloads in the process as the organisational duties of an astronaut spouse had to be balanced with the all-consuming task of preparing for one's own next mission.

Sally Ride was an early favourite for the role of FAWIS – a sharp physicist, she was also a disciplined athlete, a natural ace at the use of the shuttle's mechanical arm, and an expert in the life compartmentalisation that allows for total focus on whatever task is at hand. Resnik was to be the second American woman in space, with Seddon marked to become the third aboard STS-41E (later 41F), set for a mid-1984 launch, which was soon pushed to an August 1984 launch and then to March and ultimately April 1985, shuffled backwards by a series of bad luck occurrences that meant Seddon had to scramble to train and retrain for her flight's shifting array of missions and priorities.

That flight, STS-51-D, while on the docket it looked to be one of the more routine shuttle missions yet flown, ended in the world's first unscheduled spacewalk that attempted gamely, by ingenious use of a variety of at-hand materials (including a bone saw that Seddon, the resident surgeon, wielded to produce a necessary satellite-snagging component) to reinitiate a malfunctioning satellite. That flight also featured Seddon employing an onboard echocardiograph to record the world's first images of a heart grappling with the effects of space flight.

51-D turned out a good deal more exciting than anyone had anticipated, but with the *Challenger* disaster in 1986 and the subsequent payload reshuffling, it would be another six *years* until Seddon returned to space. Her next assigned mission, Spacelab Life Sciences 1, featured an array of biological studies that had to take a back seat in the flight rotation to the paying customers who had been waiting two and three years for NASA to place their satellites in promised orbit. In the meantime, Seddon prepared for that mission, served in a number of different administrative capacities, and found an ER unit where she could keep her skills sharp in her 'spare' moments.

Launched in 1991 and 1993, the two Spacelab Life Sciences missions studied the effects of weightlessness and space travel on animal physiology. How much harder does the heart need to work to push blood through a body evolutionarily adapted to gravity? What happens to the inner ear and brain as an individual spends a week in a weightless state then returns to Earth? What is the fate of muscle growth and differentiation in a zero G environment? These are important questions to a species looking to expand beyond the comfortable expectations of its home planet, and Seddon played an important role in defining their base parameters.

The arrival of the 1990s, however, and of a political rhetoric that found easy capital in publicly advocating a heavy curtailment of NASA funding, sent the organisation Seddon had joined in a burst of youthful adventure in 1978 into a new era that featured as its lynchpin collaboration with a Russia just emerging from the shadow of the Soviet Union. For the foreseeable future, astronauts would be expected to learn Russian, and spend long periods of time training in Russia, prospects which, though perhaps tantalising to a single 20-something, were singularly less so to a 45-year-old married mother of four with 700 hours of spaceflight already under her belt, and horror stories of the operational prerogatives and norms of the Russian space programme in her ears. The Spacelab missions were concluded by 1995, with no plans for extensive science experimentation aboard the International Space Station for at least a decade thereafter. Taken in total, the universe seemed to be saying, 'You have done what you needed to do. It's all right to move on now.'

Margaret Rhea Seddon retired from NASA in 1997, and devoted herself to the development of her medical career, the writing of her memoirs, the fostering of space education, and the needs of her children and grandchildren. Hers was the first heart the world had ever seen in space, and through two decades of low-paying service to NASA in the name of science and adventure, she showed how much heart, wedded to persistence and brains, can accomplish in our lives, so short as against those of the stars, but so very full when we choose them to be.

Further Reading

Seddon's memoirs, *Go For Orbit: One of America's First Women Astronauts Finds Her Space* (2015) is a treasure trove of space-shuttle-era autobiography that serves as an interesting counterpoint to Kathryn Sullivan's *Handprints on Hubble* (2019). Sullivan and Seddon are both hyper-talented, intelligent, and driven individuals but it would be hard to find two books so different in what they choose to focus on in the sharing of their shuttle-era memories. Seddon's is a story of achieving life balance across multiple talents and priorities, Sullivan's one of long-term focus on the achieving of specific technical goals, and together they make for a delightful reading experience.

Chapter 35

Brief Portraits

Twentieth-Century Heroes

Esther Pohl Lovejoy (1869–1967)

Esther Lovejoy was the first vice president of the Medical Women's National Association, an organisation attempting in the First World War to gain officer status for women serving in the US Army Medical Corps, and served herself as a Red Cross physician in Paris during the war. She also was effective in raising funds for the American Women's Hospitals project, which provided medical support for the civilian population as a counterweight to Elsie Inglis's Scottish Women's Hospital movement, which was focused on servicing the military sector. Following the conflict, she was elected the first president of the Medical Women's International Association in 1919, which aimed at fostering international discussion of women's medical issues, particularly between those nations that had just been enemies in the war.

Ida Sophia Scudder (1870–1960)

Born in India to a medical missionary family, Ida Scudder resolved on a medical career after she witnessed three Indian women die in childbirth rather than allow male doctors to attend them and thereby violate their religious principles. In 1899, she graduated from Cornell Medical College and then returned to India, founding a clinic for women at Vellore. In 1902, she established the Mary Taber Schell Hospital, adding a nursing school in 1909, and in 1918, the Union Mission Medical School, a women's medical school that received 151 applicants in its first year of operation and continued to expand over the subsequent decades. In 1950, the Medical School, which had been renamed the Christian Medical College in 1940, became an affiliate of the University of Madras. She died in 1960 after a half century of service in the name of Indian women's medicine.

Adah Belle Thoms (1870–1943)

Adah Thoms graduated from the Lincoln Hospital and Home School of Nursing in 1905, and within two years was at the epicentre of the black nurses' movement, hosting the 1907 meeting that created the National Association of Colored Graduate Nurses (NACGN). The NACGN sought admission for black nurses into the American Nurses' Association, as well as integration into the armed forces. Thoms served as president of the organisation from 1916–1923 and during that time succeeded in persuading the American Red Cross to allow black nurses to serve in its ranks during the First World War, which led to the limited acceptance of black nurses into the army's Nurse Corps.

Ella Phillips Crandall (1871–1938)

Ella Crandall was a pioneer in the field of public health nursing. After joining the faculty at Columbia University Teachers College in 1910, she developed new courses in district nursing and community health, and was pivotal in the American Nurses Association's creation of the National Organization for Public Health Nursing in 1912, where she served as executive secretary from 1912–1920. For the last thirteen years of her life, she was the executive secretary to the Payne Fund, which financed research on how to better educate the public on health issues.

Lillian Keturah Pond Farrar (1871–1962)

In 1921, the American Gynaecological Society had precisely one female member, and she was Lillian Farrar. She did important work pushing gynaecology into the modern era, including studies in the 1920s of radium therapy as a cure for cervical cancer, of autotransfusion for gynaecological patients (in which a patient's blood is collected and stored well ahead of a procedure involving expected large blood loss, then restored after it), of the relative merits of total hysterectomies, and of the occurrence and nature of shock in gynaecological surgeries and events. In 1925, she became the first woman to serve as a governor of the American College of Surgeons.

Marcelle Lapicque (1873–1960)

For half a century, Marcelle Lapicque studied the nature of nerve impulses, often working with her husband, renowned neurophysiologist Louis Lapicque, whom she had met while they were students at the University of Paris. Her research, published in over eighty academic articles, centred around the behaviour of a nerve impulse over time, and the response of nerve impulses to different poisons and inhibitors, particularly strychnine. She was the associate director of the École Pratique des Hautes Études from 1904 to 1952.

Harriette Chick (1875–1977)

Harriette Chick's long career as a microbiologist and nutritionist included some of the early twentieth century's most important breakthroughs in relating diet to disease. Born in London, Chick was a student and later staff member at the Lister Institute from 1905 to 1945. Here, in 1908, she formulated Chick's Law, which relates the effectiveness of a disinfectant to its time in contact with the organisms it is intended to destroy. For the next ten years, she worked on developing targeted disinfectants for particular microorganisms, before switching her interest to the interactions of diet and disease, studying the role of dietary deficiencies in scurvy and beriberi, then in 1919 forming the team that discovered the role that fat-soluble vitamins (such as those in cod liver oil) and sunlight play in preventing rickets. The success of her efforts led the Lister Institute to create a new Nutrition division, of which she was named head, allowing her to continue her research into rickets and pellagra (a disease caused by niacin deficiency). Between 1932 and 1958 her nutrition group published forty-eight papers, and worked on creating standardised guidelines for vitamins A, D, and the Vitamin B complex.

Angeliki Panajiotatou (1875–1954)

A microbiologist specialising in the study of tropical diseases, Panajiotatou was also the first woman to earn a medical degree in Greece when she graduated from the University of Athens in 1897. She was subsequently hired as a lecturer at the university, only to be boycotted by the students on account of her gender. Leaving her position in Athens, she became professor of microbiology at Cairo University, where she carried out her studies in cholera and typhus until returning at last to Greece in 1938 to serve as deputy professor of Hygiene and Tropical Medicine. In 1950, she became the first woman elected to the Academy of Athens.

Emily (née Dunning) Barringer (1876–1961)

Encouraged to join Cornell University's medical programme by family friend Mary Putnam Jacobi, Dunning graduated in 1897 and earned her medical degree in 1901 from the Cornell University School of Medicine. After receiving the second-highest grade on an internship exam for Gouverneur Hospital in New York City, her application was nonetheless rejected, compelling Dunning to gather the support of community leaders for her renewed application, which was accepted. She served as New York's first woman ambulance surgeon, experience she put to use in the First World War when she organised fundraising for the purchase of a fleet of ambulances to be sent to Europe while also serving as vice-chair of the American Women's Hospitals War Service Committee of the National Medical Women's Association. In 1942, she took over the presidency of the American Medical Women's Association, which had been founded in 1915 by Bertha van Hoosen. The 1952 MGM film *The Girl in White* starring June Allyson is based on her autobiography, *Bowery to Bellevue: The Story of New York's First Woman Ambulance Surgeon.*

Sofiya Nikolaievna Lisovskaia (1876–1951)

Sofiya Lisovskaia wrote eighty-six medical articles in the fields of immunology and urology, and served as the chair of operative surgery and topographical anatomy at the Leningrad Medical Institute from 1919 to 1937, and chair of urology there from 1933–1951. Her medical degree, earned in 1911 at the St Petersburg Women's Medical Institute, was awarded for her thesis on thyroid gland transplantation, and in her later work she modified the Debre-Pareff reaction for gonorrhoea diagnosis and studied abdominal diseases that result in elevated glucose levels in the urine.

Rosalie Slaughter Morton (1876–1968)

Morton's career is not easy to briefly summarise; she achieved so much in so many different fields it is hard to know precisely what to highlight, but here's a shot. Descended from a family tradition of male doctors who in no way encouraged her to pursue the family business, Rosalie Slaughter struck out on her own, entering the Woman's Medical College of Philadelphia in 1893. In 1899, after some time at the Alumne Hospital and Dispensary, Slaughter went on a medical tour of Europe and the colonies, studying in Berlin, Vienna, Paris and London, before travelling to Bombay to study the efficacy of new anti-plague regimens. In 1909, she became the chairman of the American Medical Association's Public Health Education Committee, in which capacity she formed alliances with local women's and mother's clubs throughout the nation to create an effective and extensive web of public health education. During the First World War, she served in Serbia and Macedonia, treating wounded soldiers and gathering information about the current state of military hospitals, then returned to New York in 1917 to co-found the American Women's Hospitals movement (mentioned previously in connection with Esther Pohl Lovejoy), while also serving as first chairman of the War Service Committee. When Congress balked at the prospect of paying for a war programme centring around women physicians, Morton and Lovejoy independently raised $300,000 in ten days for the project.

After the war, Morton continued her private practice while advocating for the United States to join the League of Nations, and carried out research in arthritis and endocrinology.

Mary Breckinridge (1881–1965)

If you are a student of American history, a little alarm bell might have just gone off – 'Breckinridge, was not that the name of the vice president to one of the worst presidents in US history?' And you are correct, John Breckinridge was the VP to the truly disastrous James Buchanan, whose granddaughter was our own Mary Breckinridge. She studied nursing at New York City Hospital, graduating in 1910. After the First World War, she served in France with the American Committee for Devastated France, working to organise a steady supply of food and medical aid to pregnant and nursing women in those areas of France devastated by war. Her experience here, and later in Scotland, revealed to her the need for better organised rural public health programmes, the cause to which she devoted the rest of her career. After studying public health at Columbia University in 1921, she formed the Kentucky Committee for Mothers and Children in 1925; this evolved into the Frontier Nursing Service (FNS), funded by Breckinridge's personal inheritance. The service organised a series of nurse outposts 10 miles apart staffed by trained nurses who could travel by horseback to reach their rural patients. The FNS is still in operation (though less horse-based than one might hope), and runs six clinics in rural Kentucky, as well as the Frontier School of Midwifery and Family Nursing.

Ethel Collins Dunham (1883–1969)

Ethel Dunham, together with her life partner Martha May Eliot, has done perhaps more for the health of premature and newborn babies than any single individual this side of Icie Macy Hoobler. In 1920, she became one of the first women to join the faculty of the Yale School of Medicine, where she began her research on neonatal mortality while introducing reforms to Yale's policies for monitoring newborn children. In 1927, she was given the job of medical officer of neonatal studies for the Children's Bureau in Washington, and on the strength of her comprehensive 1933 report on neonatal morbidity and mortality to the American Pediatric Society, she was appointed director of research in child development at the United States Children's Bureau. From that position, she developed a new model of neonatal care that featured public health nurses, social workers and paediatricians working together to provide care for premature infants, and introduced new standards of care to reduce infant mortality, which were published in 1943 and again in 1948. She wrote the pamphlet *Premature Infants* to inform paediatricians about those children's particular needs, and expanded her efforts to the world stage by working with the World Health Organization from 1949 to 1951.

Louise Pearce (1885–1959)

In 1901, a fierce outbreak of African Sleeping Sickness struck Uganda, killing a quarter of a million people, and in some villages only leaving every third human being alive. In 1910, the first drug, atoxyl, was developed to treat the disease; it was effective but also had a marked tendency to cause blindness. Clearly, a better option was needed, and a decade later the team of Louise Pearce, Walter Jacobs, Wade Brown and Michael Heidelberger had developed a new arsenic-based drug, tryparsamide. Pearce, a graduate of Stanford, Boston University and Johns Hopkins, was a Rockefeller Institute researcher under the experimental pathologist Simon Flexner. He assembled the sleeping sickness team, with Jacobs and Heidelberger developing some 243 arsenic-based compounds, while Pearce and Brown developed a model for the progress of the disease and regimens for testing the effectiveness and side-effects of the 243 potential drugs.

It fell to Pearce to travel to the Congo in 1920 to test the team's drug of choice, tryparsamide. She developed the testing protocols for the drug that determined optimum dosage in humans, and found that the drug was successful in curing 80 per cent of those infected. For the next thirty years, a combination of tryparsamide and another arsenic-based drug developed at Bayer, suramin, was the standard drug regimen for combatting African sleeping sickness. Pearce also researched tryparsamide's efficacy as an anti-syphilitic drug (in which capacity it was employed until 1950), and in the 1930s and 1940s carried out programmes of cancer and viral transmission research.

Janet Kerr Aitken (1886–1982)

For the first third of her life, Janet Aitken was on track to become a world-class classical vocalist. Born in Argentina, she moved with her family to England at the age of 4, where Aitken's musical talents were encouraged, including time in Paris to study with Madame Fillunger, who had been a friend of the German composer Robert Schumann. The First World War, however, changed the course of her life, and inspired her with the desire to become a doctor. She entered the London School of Medicine for Women in 1917, and received her medical degree in 1924. She specialised in juvenile rheumatism, and particularly rheumatic heart disease, a condition that damages the valves of the heart, and from which her younger sister had died. She served from 1929 as a physician at the Kensington Supervisory Rheumatic Clinic for Children.

Helena Rosa (née Lowenfeld) Wright (1887–1982)

Helena Wright was an early figure in the British birth control movement, who worked to improve the training of medical students in birth control and sex education. After five years spent in medical missionary work in China, Wright returned to England in 1927 to find the birth control movement split into two warring camps, with Marie Stopes advocating for nurses informing women about their birth control options, and Margery Spring Rice arguing that role should be filled by gynaecologists. Wright agreed with Rice, and in 1928 accepted her offer to work as chief medical officer at the Kensington Centre, where she developed curricula that included basic contraception practices in the training of medical students. She also wrote several books over the next three decades for a popular audience on the subjects of sex and birth control.

Katharine Scott Bishop (1889–1975)

Katharine Bishop was, with Herbert Evans, the co-discoverer of Vitamin E. Working in UC Berkeley's anatomy department, the two were studying the reproductive cycle of rats, and how it responded to different dietary regimens. In 1923, they found that rats who received all of their fat from lard grew just fine, but could not reproduce due to some dietary deficiency that caused placentas and sperm-forming cells in the testes to degrade. They called the missing substance 'Factor X' and ten years later, Evans succeeded in isolating it. Bishop did not take part in the task of isolating Vitamin E, however, due to her marriage to attorney Tyndall Bishop. She returned to her work in the 1930s, studying public health issues before becoming an anaesthetist following the death of her husband.

Gertrud Hurler (1889–1965)

Gertrud Hurler is known today for her 1919 description of Hurler Syndrome, previously known as gargoylism. The genetic condition is the result of a deficiency in an enzyme that breaks down a particular polysaccharide, which goes on to build up in our cells' lysosomes, resulting in a wide array of physical effects, including clouding of the cornea, skeletal dysplasia, spinal malalignment and cognitive impairment. Most Hurler Syndrome children die by the age of 10. After reporting the cases of two infants bearing the condition, Hurler set up a private practice in 1919 which she continued to her death in 1965, while also working towards the creation of better post-natal services in Germany.

Pearl (née Luella) Kendrick (1890–1980)

Pearl Kendrick's work as a bacteriologist continues to save the lives of thousands of children every year. In 1939, the vaccine she and Grace

Eldening developed for whooping cough, a disease that killed 6,000 children annually in the United States alone, entered mass production. She then went on to develop the modern DPT immunisation shot, which combined the diphtheria, whooping cough (pertussis), and tetanus vaccinations into one single dose, and which is still a central feature of our global children's health strategy. From the 1940s to 1960s she served as a consultant for various programmes to internationally coordinate children's vaccination programmes.

Dorothy (née Stopford) Price (1890–1954)

Dorothy Price was an Irish physician whose expertise in paediatric tuberculosis was key to the introduction of the anti-tuberculotic BCG vaccine to Ireland. She was appointed as a children's specialist to the Royal City of Dublin Hospital in 1932, and by 1936 she had begun the first Irish trials of BCG in response to an alarming upswing in paediatric tuberculosis cases. She publicised the success of those trials in her 1942 book *Tuberculosis in Childhood*, which then led to the establishment of the Irish National BCG Committee in 1949. The resulting vaccination drive dramatically reduced cases of childhood tuberculosis in Ireland, though Price did not live to see the full fruition of her efforts.

Nanna Charlotta Svartz (1890–1986)

The first full professor of medicine in Sweden, Svartz was the author of over 400 medical papers and actively pursued her research interests until the age of 93. She studied gastrointestinal diseases and rheumatology. In 1938, she proposed salicylazosulfapyridine (Salazopyrin/Azulfidine) as a drug for rheumatoid arthritis, an idea that was largely ignored during her lifetime (though it was employed as a drug to combat inflammatory bowel disease) but has since been revived.

Jerusha Jhirad (1891–1984)

Born to a Jewish Indian family, Jerusha Jhirad was the first Indian woman to receive a governmental scholarship to study medicine overseas. She earned her MD from the University of London in 1919 and returned to India in

1920, where she was medical officer-in-charge at Bangalore's maternity hospital from 1921 to 1924, and at Cama Hospital (which featured in the story of Edith Pechey-Phipson) from 1929 to 1947. Elected a Justice of the Peace in 1931, she used her combined medical knowledge and political position to carry out statistical studies of maternal mortality in Bombay and advocate for sex and contraceptive education in India.

Helen Marion Macpherson Mackay (1891–1965)

Mackay was the first woman Fellow of the Royal College of Physicians, a position she earned for her work on the causes and potential cures of childhood rickets and anaemia. She studied rickets from 1919 to 1922 in Vienna as part of the Lister Institute, before returning to England to work with microbiologist Harriette Chick's group that demonstrated the efficacy of cod liver oil and sunlight in preventing rickets. While working with Chick, she noticed the prevalence of anaemia in the children under study, and resolved to make the root causes of the disease her next field of research. Her studies discovered the role iron deficiency plays in the disease, and that breastfed children were statistically less likely to develop anaemia than formula-fed children. Her results were published in 1931 and led to her induction into the Royal College of Physicians in 1934.

Jane (née Sands) Robb (1892–?)

Robb spent most of her career at Syracuse Medical School, where she served as a professor from 1931 to 1958, and carried out research in cardiac muscle physiology, cardiac electrophysiology and cardiac pathophysiology. Together with her husband, Robert Cumming Robb, she earned the bronze medal from the American Medical Society in 1935.

Cicely Delphine Williams (1893–1992)

Born in Jamaica, Cicely Williams moved to England at the age of 13 to start her British education, which ultimately resulted in her attending Oxford in 1916 with several other young women who were allowed into the university to fill the spots vacated by the young men who were serving in the First World War. Finding that positions in England were hard to come by once the men returned from war, Williams decided to specialise in tropical medicine, and began practising in Ghana in 1929. Here she noted a number of toddler age children with distended bellies who had been diagnosed with pellagra by the local doctors. She did not concur with that finding, and performed autopsies on the children to find out more about the disease, ultimately concluding that it was the result of post-weaning protein deficiency. She called the malady by its local name, kwashiorkor, and published her findings in 1933.

The medical establishment took issue with her calling their findings into question, and did their best to bury Williams's ideas, including transferring her to Malaya in 1936. Here, she found that employees of the Nestle company were posing as nurses to convince women to use the company's sweetened condensed milk in place of breast milk, leading to a rash of child mortality. Williams did not have long to combat this false information, as she was captured during the invasion of the Japanese army, and spent the next three and half years in a Japanese jail, where she was tortured, starved and confined to a cage. Returning to England after the war, she was made head of the WHO's Maternal and Child Health Division, and ultimately returned to Malaya to oversee all maternal and child care services throughout south-east Asia.

Safiye Ali (1894–1952)

Safiye Ali was Turkey's first woman doctor; she was educated in Germany during the First World War and returned to Turkey in 1923 where she was granted a medical licence. She had significant difficulty finding private clients in her first years of practice due to lack of support among other members of the medical community, and her insistence on being paid at the same rate as male doctors for her services. She worked to spread information about modern infant nutrition practices throughout Turkey, and organised teams of nurses to visit new mothers' homes and teach them about the nutritional and sanitary needs of their children.

Dorothy Russell (1895–1983)

Dorothy Russell was an expert in the pathologies of the nervous system, specialising in tumours of the nervous system and the build-up of fluids in the cavities of the brain – known as hydrocephalus. She was the author of the classic texts *Histological Technique for Intracranial Tumours* (1939), *Observations on the Pathology of Hydrocephalus* (1949), and *Pathology of Tumours of the Nervous System* (1959).

Ruth Lundeen Memmler (1900–?)

Ruth Memmler was a teacher at Los Angeles County Hospital (1941–1945), and professor at East Los Angeles College (1945–1965) who was interested in the development of new curricula for the training of nurses, to which end she wrote two successful textbooks: *The Human Body in Health and Disease* (1959) and *Structure and Function of the Human Body* (1970), which are at present on their fourteenth and twelfth editions, respectively.

Hattie Alexander (1901–1968)

Hattie Alexander began her career in 1932 at Columbia University's Department of Pediatrics, where she remained until her retirement. Here she conducted foundational research on meningitis that established the utility of precipitin tests for meningitis prognoses, and the 75 per cent efficacy of an anti-pneumonia serum for curing infants with influenzal meningitis. She also developed an antiserum for *Haemophilus influenzae* meningitis that combined rabbit serum with sulphur drugs that knocked *Haemophilus* mortality rates from 100 to just under 25 per cent. The later addition of antibodies to the treatment plan lowered mortality rates further still. While performing these studies, Alexander noted diminished efficacy to some antibiotic treatments, and hypothesised that random genetic mutations in the bacteria were the root cause of the phenomenon, thereby contributing to the early development of antibiotic resistance theory.

Dorothy Hansine Andersen (1901–1963)

In 1938, Dorothy Andersen published an article identifying and describing a new disease which she called cystic fibrosis. From 1935 to 1938 she had been studying patients who suffered from coeliac disease, a genetic condition that causes the body to produce autoantibodies in response to the presence of gluten, which go on to affect different organs, particularly the small intestine. In performing autopsies of patients diagnosed with coeliac disease, she noticed the presence of cysts and scarring on the pancreas that were also present in the lungs. She developed diagnostic tests for the new disease, but the determination of its cause would have to wait for the genetic techniques of a later generation. Thanks to her efforts in diagnosis and treatment, cystic fibrosis patients, who rarely lived past childhood, began surviving into young adulthood, and Andersen devoted her last paper, in 1959, to a study of those individuals.

Lin Qiaozhi (1901–1983)

Known as the 'Mother of Ten Thousand Babies', Lin Qiaozhi was a moderniser of Chinese gynaecology who, after study in Europe, managed to continue her career through the manifold ideological twists and turns of mid-century China. She served on the staff at Peking Union Medical College from 1929 to 1983, with a six-year interlude at Zhonghe Hospital from 1942 to 1948, and fulfilled not only the numerous professional committee responsibilities that are the lot of many doctors in Communist China, but carried out research (publishing under the name Kim Ha Ti) in neonatal haemolytic disorders, diseases of the female pelvis, and foetal breathing.

Marthe Louise Vogt (1903–2003)

Marthe Vogt arrived in England in 1935, fleeing the rise of the Nazi party in her native Germany, and there began her work with Sir Henry Dale on acetylcholine's role in voluntary motor nerve activity, which won Dale a Nobel Prize and her a mention in his Nobel Prize speech. Later, she made a more in-depth study of acetylcholine with William Feldberg which, in 1948, provided evidence for the chemical's role as a neurotransmitter.

Myra Adele Logan (1908–1977)

Myra Logan was the first woman surgeon to perform open-heart surgery, and only the ninth person in the world to perform any type of bypass surgery. She was born in Jim Crow-era Tuskegee, Alabama, and went on to a residency at Harlem Hospital where she not only performed her history-making bypass operation in 1943, but also worked for the development of new antibiotic treatments. She was a pioneer in the use of Aureomycin and Puromycin, and developed X-ray techniques to allow the distinguishing of healthy and cancerous breast tissues.

Virginia Apgar (1909–1974)

Apgar's name is probably familiar to most people from the Apgar Score she developed in 1952, which gave doctors and nurses a fast set of diagnostic criteria to evaluate the general health of newborn children at one minute after birth. She went back to school in 1959 to earn a master's degree in Public Health at Johns Hopkins University, then spent the rest of her career with the March of Dimes, which had developed out of the great polio epidemic of the early twentieth century and which Apgar employed as a platform to shine a light on important public health issues, including the use of Rh testing to prevent maternal antibodies from attacking foetal red blood cells; universal rubella vaccination as a means of fighting the great 1964 rubella outbreak that infected over 12 million individuals in the United States; problems associated with premature births; and greater knowledge of birth defects and their different health care requirements.

Selected Bibliography

Reference Works & General Histories

Abir-Am, Pnina G. and Dorinda Outram, ed., *Uneasy Careers and Intimate Lives: Women in Science, 1789–1979.* (Rutgers University, 1987).

Abram, Ruth J. ed., *'Send Us a Lady Physician': Women Doctors in America, 1835–1920.* (W. W. Norton, 1985).

Atwater, Edward, *Women Medical Doctors in the United States Before the Civil War: A Biographical Dictionary.* (University of Rochester Press, 2016).

Brittain, Vera, *The Women at Oxford: A Fragment of History.* (Macmillan Company, 1960).

Campbell, Olivia, *Women in White Coats: How the First Women Doctors Changed the World of Medicine.* (Park Row Books, 2021).

Carrell, Jennifer Lee, *The Speckled Monster: A Historical Tale of Battling Smallpox.* (Plume, 2004).

Cole, Jonathan R., *Fair Science: Women in the Scientific Community.* (Free Press, 1979).

Creese, Mary R. S., *Ladies in the Laboratory? American and British Women in Science, 1800–1900: A Survey of Their Contributions to Research.* (Scarecrow Press, 1998).

Dodge, Bertha S., *The Story of Nursing.* (Little, Brown and Company, 1954).

Fara, Patricia, *A Lab of One's Own: Science and Suffrage in the First World War.* (Oxford University Press, 2018).

Haines, Catharine M. C., *International Women In Science: A Biographical Dictionary to 1950.* (ABC-Clio, 2001).

LeClair, Mary K., Justin D. White, and Susan Keeter, *Three Nineteenth-Century Women Doctors: Elizabeth Blackwell, Mary Walker, and Sarah Loguen Fraser.* (Hofmann Press, 2007).

Levin, Miriam R., *Defining Women's Scientific Enterprise. Mount Holyoke Faculty and the Rise of American Science.* (University Press of New England, 2005).

Lipinska, Mélanie, *Histoire des Femmes Médecins: Depuis L'antiquité jusqu'a Nos Jours.* (Librarie G. Jacques & C., 1900).

Marland, Hilary ed., *The Art of Midwifery: Early Modern Midwives in Europe.* (Routledge, 1993).

Marshall, Clara, *The Woman's Medical College of Pennsylvania: An Historical Outline.* (P. Blakiston Son & Company, 1897).

McGrayne, Sharon Bertsch, *Nobel Prize Women in Science: Their Struggles, and Momentous Discoveries.* (Joseph Henry Press, 1993).

More, Ellen S., *Restoring the Balance: Women Physicians and the Profession of Medicine, 1850–1995.* Harvard University Press, 1999).

More, Ellen S., Elizabeth Fee, and Manon Parry, *Women Physicians and the Cultures of Medicine.* (Johns Hopkins University Press, 2009).

Ogilvie, Marilyn Bailey, *Women in Science: Antiquity through the Nineteenth Century. A Biographical Dictionary with Annotated Bibliography.* (MIT Press, 1986).

Ogilvie, Marilyn and Joy Harvey, ed., *The Biographical Dictionary of Women in Science: Pioneering Lives from Ancient Times to the Mid-Twentieth Century.* 2 vols. (New York, Routledge, 2000).

O'Hern, Elizabeth Moot, *Profiles of Pioneer Women Scientists.* (Acropolis Books Ltd, 1985).

Oshinsky, David M., *Polio: An American Story.* (Oxford University Press, 2005).

Perronne, Bobette, H. Henrietta Stockel, and Victoria Krueger, *Medicine Women, Curanderas, and Women Doctors.* (University of Oklahoma, 1989).

Rossiter, Margaret W., *Women Scientists in America: Volume I: Struggles and Strategies to 1940.* (Johns Hopkins University Press, 1982).

— *Women Scientists in America: Volume 2: Before Affirmative Action: 1940–1972.* (Johns Hopkins University Press, 1998).

— *Women Scientists in America: Volume 3: Forging a New World Since 1972.* (Johns Hopkins University Press, 2012).

Stapp, Cheryl Anne, *Disaster & Triumph: Sacramento Women, Gold Rush through the Civil War.* (2012).

Whaley, Leigh, *Women and the Practice of Medical Care in Early Modern Europe, 1400–1800.* (Palgrave Macmillan, 2011).

Yost, Edna, *American Women of Nursing.* (J. B. Lippincott Company, 1947).

— *American Women of Science.* (Frederick A. Stokes Company, 1943).

— *Women of Modern Science.* (Dodd, Mead and Company, 1966).

Biographies & Memoirs

Anderson, Louisa Garrett, *Elizabeth Garrett Anderson: 1836–1917.* (Faber and Faber Limited, 1939).

Baker, Jean H., *Margaret Sanger: A Life of Passion.* (Hill and Wang, 2011).

Barré-Sinoussi, Françoise, *Pour un Monde sans SIDA: Un Combat Partagé.* (Albin Michel, 2012).

Barringer, Emily Dunning, *Bowery to Bellevue: The Story of New York's First Woman Ambulance Surgeon.* (Norton, 1950).

Bek, Anna. Transl. Anne D. Rassweiler, *The Life of a Russian Woman Doctor: A Siberian Memoir, 1869–1954.* (Indiana University Press, 2004).

Bittel, Carla, *Mary Putnam Jacobi and the Politics of Medicine in Nineteenth Century America.* (University of North Carolina, 2009).

Blackwell, Elizabeth, *Pioneer Work in Opening the Medical Profession to Women.* (1895).

Bluemel, Elinor, *Florence Sabin: Colorado Woman of the Century.* (University of Colorado Press).

Boyd, Julia, *The Excellent Doctor Blackwell. The Life of the First Woman Physician.* (Thistle Publishing, 2013).

Breckinridge, Mary, *Wide Neighborhoods: A Story of the Frontier Nursing Service.* (University Press of Kentucky, 1981).

Brinkschulte, Eva, and Eva Labouvie, *Dorothea Christiana Erxleben: Weibliche Gelehrsamkeit und medizinische Profession seit dem 18. Jahrhundert.* (Mitteldeutscher Verlag, 2006).

Caldicott, Helen, *A Desperate Passion: An Autobiography.* (W. W. Norton and Company, 1996).

Colwell, Rita, *A Lab of One's Own: One Woman's Personal Journey Through Sexism in Science.* (Simon & Schuster, 2020).

Cornell, Virginia, *Doc Susie: The True Story of a Country Physician in the Colorado Rockies.* (Carpinteria, Manifest Publications, 1991).

Craddock, Sally, *Retired, Except on Demand: The Life of Dr Cicely Williams.* (Green College, 1983).

Dall, Caroline Healey, *The Life of Dr Anandibai Joshee, a Kinswoman of the Pundita Ramabai.* (Roberts Brothers, 1888).

Daniels, Anna K., *It's Never Too Late To Love.* (Pyramid Books, 1953).

Dash, Joan, *A Life of One's Own: Three Gifted Women and the Men They Married.* (Harper and Row, 1973).

Davis, Elizabeth. ed. Jane Williams, *Betsy Cadwaladyr: A Balaclava Nurse.* (Honno Classics, 2007).

Epler, Percy Harold, *The Life of Clara Barton.* (New York, Arno Press, 1980).

Gelbart, Nina Rattner, *The King's Midwife: A History and Mystery of Madame du Coudray.* (University of California Press, 1998).

Glenn, Myra C., *Dr Harriot Kezia Hunt: Nineteenth-Century Physician and Women's Rights Advocate.* (University of Massachusetts Press, 2018).

Green, Monica H., *The Trotula: An English Translation of the Medieval Compendium of Women's Medicine.* (University of Pennsylvania, 2001).

Hellstedt, Leone McGregor, *Women Physicians of the World: Autobiographies of Medical Pioneers*. (Hemisphere Publishing, 1978).

Hunt, Harriot K., *Glances and Glimpses; or, Fifty Years Social, Including Twenty Years Professional Life.* (Boston, J. P. Jewett and Co, 1856).

Hutton, Isabel, *Memories of a Doctor in War & Peace.* (Heinemann, 1960).

Jensen, Kimberly, *Oregon's Doctor to the World: Esther Pohl Lovejoy and a Life in Activism.* (University of Washington Press, 2012).

Koven, Suzanne, *Letter to a Young Female Physician.* (W. W. Norton and Company, 2021).

Leneman, Leah, *Elsie Inglis: Founder of Battlefront Hospitals Run Entirely by Women.* (NMS Publishing, 1998).

Lovejoy, Esther Pohl, *House of the Good Neighbor*. 1919.

Lutzker, Edythe, *Edith Pechey-Phipson MD, The Story of England's Foremost Pioneering Woman Doctor*. (Exposition Press, 1973).

Manton, Jo, *Elizabeth Garrett Anderson.* (E. P. Dutton and Company, 1965).

Morton, Rosalie Slaughter, *A Woman Surgeon: The Life and Work of Rosalie Slaughter Morton.* (Frederick A. Stokes, 1937).

— *A Doctor's Holiday in Iran*. (Funk and Wagnalls, 1940).

Nightingale, Florence. Ed. Sue M. Goldie, *Florence Nightingale: Letters from the Crimea.* (Mandolin, 1997).

Nimura, Janice P., *The Doctors Blackwell: How Two Pioneering Sisters Brought Medicine to Women and Women to Medicine.* (W. W. Norton & Company, 2022).

Oates, Stephen B., *Woman of Valor: Clara Barton and the Civil War.* (Free Press, 1995).

Parsons, Emily Elizabeth, *Fearless Purpose: Memoir of Emily Elizabeth Parsons*. (Little Brown and Company, 1880).

Phelan, Mary Kay, *Probing the Unknown: The Story of Dr Florence Sabin.* (Thomas Y. Crowell Company, 1969).

Pollack, Linda, *With faith and Physic: The Life of a Tudor Gentlewoman, Lady Grace Mildmay, 1552–1620.* (London, Collins and Brown, 1993).

Rao, Yi, Daqing Zhang, and Runhong Li, *Tu Youyou and the Discovery of Artemisinin.* (World Scientific, 2017).

Roberts, Shirley, *Sophia Jex-Blake: A Woman Pioneer in Nineteenth-Century Medical Reform.* (Routledge, 1993).

Seddon, Rhea, *Go For Orbit: One of America's First Astronauts Finds Her Space.* (Your Space Press, 2015).

Sharp, Jane. Ed. Elaine Hobby, *The Midwives Book: Or the Whole Art of Midwifery Discovered.* (Oxford University Press, 1999).

Singer, Joy Daniels, *My Mother, The Doctor.* (E. P. Dutton & Co, 1970).

Straus, Eugene, *Rosalyn Yalow: Nobel Laureate. Her Life and Work in Medicine.* (Plenum Trade, 1998).

Thomas, Vivien T., *Partners of the Heart: Vivien Thomas and his Work with Alfred Blalock.* (University of Pennsylvania Press, 1985).

Tiburtius, Franziska, *Erinnerungen einer Achtzigjahrigen.* (Scjwetschke & Sohn, 1923).

Todd, Margaret, *The Life of Sophia Jex-Blake.* (Macmillan and Company, 1918).

Tuchman, Arleen, *Science has no Sex: The Life of Marie Zakrzewska.* (University of North Carolina Press, 2006).

Van Hoosen, Bertha, *Petticoat Surgeon.* (Kessinger Publishing, 2010).

Wilkie, Katherine E. and Elizabeth R. Moseley, *Frontier Nurse: Mary Breckinridge.* (New York, Messner, 1969).

Willett, Jo, *The Pioneering Life of Mary Wortley Montagu: Scientist and Feminist.* (Pen and Sword Books, 2021).

Woodham-Smith, Cecil, *Florence Nightingale: 1820–1910.* (McGraw-Hill Book Company, 1951).

Wu, Judy Tzu-Chun, *Doctor Mom Chung of the Fair-Haired Bastards: The Life of a Wartime Celebrity.* (University of California Press, 2005).

Yount, Lisa, *Alfred Blalock, Helen Taussig & Vivien Thomas: Mending Children's Hearts.* (Chelsea House, 2012).

Index